Hearing impairment

Hearing impairment

A guide for people with auditory
handicaps and those concerned
with their care and rehabilitation

Kenneth Lysons

Woodhead-Faulkner · Cambridge

Published by Woodhead-Faulkner Limited
Fitzwilliam House, 32 Trumpington Street, Cambridge CB2 1QY

First published 1984

ISBN 0 85941 230 X (cased)
ISBN 0 85941 246 6 (paperback)

Library of Congress Cataloging in Publication Data
Lysons, Kenneth.
 Hearing impairment.

 Includes index.
  1. Hearing disorders. I. Title.
 RF290.L94 1984 617.8′9 84-1525
 ISBN 0-85941-230-X
 ISBN 0-85941-246-6 (pbk.)

Designed by Geoff Green
Typeset by Hands Fotoset, Leicester
Printed in Great Britain by
St Edmundsbury Press, Bury St Edmunds, Suffolk

To
Edith Mary Lysons
Mary Plackett

Contents

Acknowledgements

This book could not have been written without the help of many people. It would be impossible to mention by name all those who have contributed to the book, but I owe a special debt to three people.

Mary Plackett, the Librarian of the Royal National Institute for the Deaf (RNID), has shown unwearying patience in dealing with numerous requests for assistance. In dedicating the book partly to her, I am making a very inadequate token of appreciation, not only of my indebtedness to Miss Plackett's help, but to all librarians. Librarians, sadly, are not always included in the acknowledgements page, let alone in the dedication, but what would any serious writer do without them?

Arthur Verney of the British Deaf Association (BDA) gave practical help and encouragement, and I am once more indebted both to his kindness and the ready help I received from all members of the BDA staff, especially Robert Peckford and Susanne Turfus.

Ian Kershaw, Principal Welfare Officer of the St Helens Society for the Deaf, took an interest in the book from its inception, and was indefatigable in suggesting possible contacts and sources of information.

Others who have given special help include Dr Denzil Brooks, Dr J. C. Denmark, Mr M. C. Martin, Miss Rosemary McCall, Dr S. D. G. Stephens, and Mr H. Zalin, FRCS.

I am indebted to the following for permission to include copyright material: S. Karger for permission to include the Social Hearing Handicap Index by Ewartsen and Birk-Nielsen as published in *Audiology*, Vol. 12, 1973; Aram Glorig, MD, and the

American Speech-Language Hearing Association for the Scale for the Self Assessment of Hearing published in the *Journal of Speech and Hearing Disorders* Vol. 29, (1964); the Editor, the *Journal of Auditory Research* for the inclusion of the Hearing Measurement Scale by Noble and Atherley. The Editor of the *British Journal of Audiology* kindly allowed me to use some material from his journal, and the Controller of Her Majesty's Stationery Office allowed the use of some items from Department of Health and Social Security publications. Granada Publications kindly gave permission to use some material from my earlier book *How To Cope With Hearing Loss*.

Finally, I would record my thanks to Margaret Reid, Rita Leyland and Brenda Walker, who competently turned manuscript into typescript.

C. K. L.

Chapter 1

The meaning, categories and incidence of hearing impairment

This book is written for all who wish to understand hearing impairment and the assistance available to those with a hearing loss. Whilst not a textbook, it should prove informative to physiological measurement technicians (audiology), disablement resettlement officers, hearing aid dispensers and hearing therapists, health visitors, nurses, social workers and speech therapists who, as part of their training, are required to obtain a knowledge of hearing impairment. Those within the community who are likely to encounter hearing impaired persons, such as general practitioners, ministers of religion, the police, personnel officers and staffs of employment and social security offices, may also find the book useful as a source of quick reference. A third group comprises hearing impaired persons themselves, their friends and their families.

After reading this book the reader should be able to:

1 State the principal types of hearing impairment, their causes and consequences.
2 Understand what is meant by sound and how we hear it.
3 Describe how hearing impairment in children and adults can be detected, diagnosed and measured.
4 Appreciate some of the possible psychological and social consequences of pre-lingual or acquired hearing impairment.
5 Explain and evaluate the communication methods used by hearing impaired persons.
6 Indicate what assistance is available to pre-lingually deaf, deafened and hard of hearing persons through the statutory and voluntary agencies, especially those relating to education, health and social work.

1

7   State what types of hearing and other aids are available to assist hearing impaired persons with their disability.

Before proceeding further, however, the term 'hearing impairment' should be clarified.

What is hearing impairment?

The words 'impairment', 'disability' and 'handicap' are often used interchangeably. When assessing individual needs and how to meet them it is useful to define these terms more precisely.[1]

Impairment is an anatomical, pathological or psychological loss or defect describable in diagnostic or symptomatic terms.

Disability is a limitation of performance in one or more activities which are generally accepted as essential basic components of daily living such that partial or complete inability to perform them necessitates a degree of dependence on a compensatory aid and/or another person.

Handicap comprises the disadvantages or restrictions of activity experienced by an individual as a result of the impairment or disability.

These distinctions become clearer when applied to a specific case. Mr X is a bank clerk with a progressive hearing loss. The defective hearing is his *impairment*. He has difficulty in hearing normal conversation so that he cannot deal with customers. This is his *disability*. Because of his disability, X's promotion opportunities are restricted. He is therefore *handicapped*. If X can largely overcome his hearing loss by using a hearing aid he will have an impairment but not necessarily a disability. The hearing aid, however, makes his impairment visible and this may still prejudice his chances of promotion. Although the disability has been overcome, he is still handicapped.

'Environment' is another term to be considered. Our environment is the external world that surrounds us. We make contact with our environment through our five senses. Any hearing impairment affects one of the most important ways in which we can receive information from the external environment. Hearing impairment can therefore be defined as 'any loss of hearing varying from slight to profound, affecting, according to its time of onset and severity, the ability of an individual to make normal auditory contact with his or her environment'.

The classification of hearing impairment

In everyday speech, the term 'deaf' is used for all types of hearing impairment irrespective of the severity of the loss or its time of onset. Even the *Shorter Oxford Dictionary* defines the word 'deaf' as 'lacking or defective in the sense of hearing'. Four factors that must be considered when classifying hearing impairment are its severity, type, time of onset and development of speech and language.

Severity of impairment

A fundamental distinction is between persons who are *deaf* and *hard of hearing*. The former have been defined as 'those in whom the sense of hearing is non-functional for the ordinary purposes of life'. The latter are 'those in whom the sense of hearing, although defective, is functional with or without a hearing aid'.[2] To be deaf means to have no usable hearing and is therefore a more severe impairment than to be hard of hearing which implies some degree of usable hearing even though amplification by means of a hearing aid may be necessary. This distinction must be kept constantly in mind since, as will be shown later, the problems of the deaf are very different from those of the hard of hearing.

For educational purposes a distinction was formerly made between *deaf* and *partially hearing* (see p. 4). Hearing loss may also be categorised as *slight, moderate, severe* or *total*. As shown in Chapter 4 it is possible to quantify these terms.

Type of impairment

Hearing impairment can also be classified according to the part(s) of the ear where the loss is located. The terms *conductive loss, perceptive* or *sensorineural loss* and *mixed loss* are explained in Chapter 3.

Time of onset

Hearing impairment may be *congenital*, i.e. occurring at or before birth, or *acquired* or *adventitious* when the loss arises after birth. From the standpoints of education and rehabilitation, the distinction between *pre-lingual* and *post-lingual* deafness is particularly important. The former relates to 'the condition of persons whose deafness was present at birth or occurred at an age prior to the development of speech and language'. The latter refers to 'the condition of persons whose deafness occurred at an age following the spontaneous acquisition of speech and language'.[3]

The word *deafened* is sometimes used to describe a person previously with normal hearing who through such causes as disease, accident or exposure to loud noise has acquired a severe or total hearing loss. Where the loss has occurred suddenly the term *traumatically deafened* is sometimes used.

The development of speech and language

This classification, closely related to the time of onset, is used to determine the most appropriate educational methods for a hearing impaired child. The Handicapped Pupils and Special Schools Amending Regulations 1962 classified pupils with impaired hearing into two categories, defined as follows:

deaf pupils, that is to say, pupils with impaired hearing who require education by methods suitable for pupils with little or no naturally acquired speech or language; partially hearing pupils, that is to say, pupils with impaired hearing whose development of speech and language, even if retarded, is following a normal pattern, and who require for their education special arrangements or facilities though not necessarily all the educational methods used for deaf pupils.

The Report of the Committee of Enquiry into the Education of Handicapped Children and Young People (Warnock) recommended that the statutory categories of all pupils requiring special educational treatment should be abolished.

DHSS classification

The Department of Health and Social Security (DHSS) requires local authorities to keep registers of handicapped persons who apply to them for assistance. The basis on which 'persons with a disabling loss of hearing' are entered on such registers is 'according to the individual's present condition and needs rather than the origin of his ability'.[4] Individuals may be registered under one of the following headings:

Deaf without speech. Those who have no useful hearing and whose normal means of communication is by signs, finger-spelling or writing.

Deaf with speech. Those who (even with a hearing aid) have little or no useful hearing but whose normal method of communication is by speech and lip-reading.

The hard of hearing. Those who (with or without a hearing aid) have some useful hearing and whose normal method of communication is by speech, listening and lip-reading.

Categories of hearing impaired persons

'Hearing impairment' is a generic term covering a wide spectrum of both deaf and hard of hearing people of varying ages, conditions and needs. The following list is by no means exhaustive.

1   Pre-school deaf or partially hearing children.
2   Deaf or partially hearing children of school age.
3   Deaf or partially hearing children with other impairments or handicaps.
4   Adolescent deaf or hard of hearing young persons.
5   Adult deaf persons without speech.
6   Adult deaf persons with speech.
7   Traumatically deafened persons.
8   Hard of hearing persons.
9   Deaf-blind or blind-deaf persons.

Some hearing impaired persons have special short-term needs such as the person with a severe hearing loss who is admitted to hospital for a limited period. With others, such as an elderly hearing impaired person who is admitted to residential accommodation, the need for help in coping with the disability of defective hearing will remain throughout life.

In the above subheading the most important word is *persons*. Labelling hearing impaired people as *the* deaf or *the* hard of hearing should be avoided for two reasons. Firstly, it is depersonalising as the individual is reduced to a 'client', 'case' or member of an impaired 'class' which implies that he is less than a normal person. Secondly, whilst a hearing impaired person has problems common to others with approximately the same type and degree of hearing loss, he has also other problems specific to his own needs and environment.

The incidence of hearing impairment

Statistics relating to hearing impaired children in England who are receiving special educational treatment are prepared by the Department of Education and Science (DES). For other parts of the United Kingdom, separate statistics are prepared by the Scottish, Welsh and Northern Ireland Departments of Education. Table 1.1 shows the number of deaf and partially hearing children in England who, in January 1981, were receiving education.

Table 1.1. Number of deaf and partially hearing children in England receiving education in January 1981 (DES)

1   Number of deaf or partially hearing children in England receiving education in special schools, independent schools, designated special classes in secondary schools; boarded in homes; receiving education in hospitals, other groups or at home; and awaiting admission to special school in January 1981.
2   Prevalence of above per 10,000 of total school population.

Region	Total school population	Deaf (1)	(2)	Partially hearing (1)	(2)
North	600,775	237	3.95	313	5.21
Yorkshire and Humberside	951,266	397	4.17	424	4.46
East Midlands	728,721	329	4.51	317	4.35
East Anglia	341,581	86	2.52	170	4.98
Greater London	1,144,215	659	5.76	772	6.75
Other South East	1,887,938	861	4.56	1,225	6.49
South West	773,392	238	3.08	453	5.86
West Midlands	1,026,105	318	3.10	510	4.97
North West	1,226,132	346	2.73	845	6.67
TOTAL ENGLAND	8,720,125	3,471	3.98	5,029	5.77

Note: Handicapped children placed in ordinary classes in ordinary schools are not included in the above figures.

No statistics exist, however, for hearing impaired children attending ordinary schools and classes. As Shepherd[5] points out, these

include children whose hearing impairment is recognised and who need support from a peripatetic teacher or simply a front seat in the classroom; and also those who may not be regarded as hearing impaired but who suffer from fluctuating middle ear disorders which they may outgrow.

The prevalence rate for profound pre-lingual deafness in children is thought to be between 0.8 and 1.5 per 1,000 live births.[6]

For adults, the most comprehensive survey of the incidence was that conducted by the Central Office of Information in 1947 for the Medical Research Council to ascertain the number of hearing aids likely to be required for free loan under the National Health Service (NHS). This survey based on a stratified random sample of the civilian population over 16 years defined hearing ability in seven categories, as shown in Table 1.2.

Table 1.2 Definition of hearing ability 1947 (COI)

Category	Term	Criterion	Estimated numbers
7	Deaf mutes	Those who became deaf in early life and learned speech by special means	15,000
6	Totally deaf	Person cannot hear speech at all but had learned speech by normal means before becoming deaf	30,000
5	Deaf to all natural speech	Person has difficulty in hearing loudly spoken speech but can hear amplified speech by means of a hearing aid or trumpet	70,000
4	Hard of hearing	Person has difficulty in hearing normal direct speech but can hear loudly spoken speech	790,000
3	Hard of hearing	Person has difficulty in hearing in any part of a theatre or in group conversation but can hear speech at short range without aid	860,000
			1,765,000

Categories 1 and 2 referred respectively to those who 'can hear all normal speech in any part of theatre/church without aid' and 'have one defective ear, but who can hear all normal speech in any part of theatre/church or in group conversation without aid'.

In 1976 the Statistics and Research Division of the DHSS updated the 1947 figures to reflect changes in the age distribution of the population. An estimate of the prevalance rates for children was also made. The results are given in Tables 1.3 and 1.4.

For the purpose of the tables 'very severe impairment' is defined as 'inability to hear speech at all even with amplifica-

Table 1.3 Estimate of number of hearing impaired people aged 16 and over living in the community

Class	1975 000s	1947 000s
Very severe impairment	62	45
Other impairments	2,298	1,720
Totals	2,360	1,765

Table 1.4 Estimates of prevalence of deafness and of hearing impairment for children under age 16 in Great Britain.

Class	Prevalence rate per 1000	No. pre-school 000s	No. school age 000s
Very severe impairment	1.6	6.2	15.4
Other impairments	11.0	41.9	106.1
Totals	12.6	48.1	121.5

tion'. 'Other impairments' covers 'all other hearing defects down to and including difficulty in hearing in public places or in group conversation'.

Two other sources published by the DHSS are the *Annual Registers of Handicapped Persons* and details of the issue and replacement of government hearing aids.[4] The former compiled from the local authority registers of handicapped persons referred to already are incomplete, since registration is voluntary. The latter provides a far from complete indication of people requiring an aid to maintain social adequacy.

In 1980 the figures for England only were:

First issues	*Exchanges*	*Replacements*	*Total*
126,185	49,178	228,168	403,531

Independent surveys also provide useful information. A study[7] accompanied by audiometric tests of 253 people aged 70 and over and living at home showed a high prevalence of impairment:

60% were significantly hearing impaired in both ears.
69% of those aged 75 were hearing impaired.
82% of those aged 80 were hearing impaired.
84% of those aged 85 were hearing impaired.
54% suffered from tinnitus.
14% of the total sample were impaired in one ear only.

Statistics of hearing impairment are essential for community planning but should never blind us to the needs of the individual hearing impaired person.

References

1 The definitions have been adapted from those offered by Garrard in *Impairment, Disability and Handicap*, Lees and Shaw (Eds), Heinemann, 1974.
2 *Definitions of the Committee on Nomenclature representing the Conference of Executives of American Schools for the Deaf*, 1937.
3 Definitions from Moores, D. F., *Educating the Deaf: Psychology, Principles and Practices*, Houghton Mifflin Company, 1978.
4 Ministry of Health Circular 25/61 and subsequent revisions.
5 Shepherd, L. 'The Availability of Statistics relating to Deafness in the United Kingdom', *British Journal of Audiology*, 12, 1978, pp.3–8.
6 DHSS Advisory Committee on Services for Hearing Impaired People. *Report of Sub-committee appointed to consider the Role of Social Services in the Care of the Deaf of all Kinds*, June 1977, p.4.
7 Herbst, K. G. and Humphrey, C. 'Prevalence of Hearing Impairment in the Elderly living at Home', *Journal of Royal College of General Practitioners*, March 1981.

Chapter 2

Sound and hearing

Every day we are exposed to sound of many kinds which may serve a variety of purposes. Sound such as music provides aesthetic experience. As speech, sound is the most important form of human communication. A ringing doorbell or a wailing siren can alert. A motor mechanic listening to an engine or a doctor detecting a heart murmur are both using sound for diagnostic purposes. Loud or persistent sound such as a radio at full volume or a dripping tap can annoy. Excessive sound can damage the sensitive instrument intended for its reception – the human ear.

What is sound?

Sound originates in the vibration of a body. Sometimes, as with the quivering prongs of a tuning fork struck against a hard object, the vibrations can be seen. Place your fingers on your throat as you talk and the vibrating chords can be felt. Since sound will not pass through a vacuum it must be conducted through some medium. This medium is usually the air although the material medium for transmission may take a solid or liquid form. From the sound source the vibrations will result in sound waves similar to the ripples produced by throwing a stone into a pond.

Although sound waves have different forms, a pure-tone note (one that is restricted to a single frequency), such as that emitted by a tuning fork, may be represented diagramatically as in Fig. 2.1.

When a tuning fork is caused to vibrate, particles of air are first compressed or pushed outwards so that they collide with neighbouring particles to form a compression. A chain reaction is thus set up similar to railway wagons pushing each other forward in a shunting operation. In between the particles spread out again and expansion takes place.

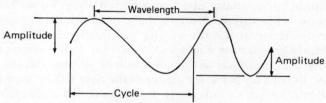

Fig. 2.1 Characteristics of sound

From the standpoint of this book the most important attributes of a sound wave are its frequency (pitch) and intensity.

The *frequency* or *pitch* of a sound wave is normally equal to the number of vibrations, or complete cycles of compression and expansion, per second. The distance from the crest of one wave to the crest of the next is known as *the wavelength*.

The technical term for 'cycles per second' is Hertz (Hz). If, in one second, a sound results in 2,000 compressions and expansions, it has a frequency of 2,000 Hz. A young adult with normal hearing has an audible range from about 15 Hz to 20,000 Hz. Sounds below and above this audible range are described as infrasonic and ultrasonic respectively. As we grow older, capacity to hear the higher frequencies diminishes. Few persons over 60 years can hear tones higher than 10,000 Hz. This loss has little practical significance, however, since the all important speech frequencies fall between 250 Hz to 4,000 Hz.

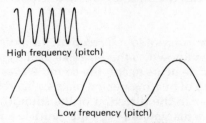

High frequency (pitch)

Low frequency (pitch)

Fig. 2.2 Frequency or pitch

In speech the majority of English vowel sounds are medium to low frequency. Consonants cover a wider frequency range. The consonants in *m, n, ng, l, d, b, j* are all low frequency; conversely *t* and *f* are over 3,000 Hz while *s* and *th* are the highest speech sounds of all.

Intensity is the energy put into the sound by its source, e.g. the force with which a tuning fork is struck. This is shown by the amplitude or maximum displacement of a wave. Loudness and intensity, while different, are related since loudness depends on intensity. If we strike the tuning fork gently a wave of low amplitude or soft note will result. When the fork is struck more forcibly the amplitude of the wave will be greater and the note louder. In both cases the frequency of the note will be the same.

The loudness of sound clearly decreases with distance from its source. Under ideal conditions sound intensity is inversely proportional to the square of the distance from the sound source. In simple terms this means that if you are in the open air listening to a person standing 2ft away and he moves to a distance of 4ft his voice will sound not half but only one quarter as loud as previously. Hearing impaired persons should therefore discover the approximate distance at which conversation can be heard under different conditions such as in a quiet room or out of doors and endeavour to keep within this range of the speaker.

The ear and hearing

Three conditions must exist for a sound to be heard:
1   A sound source consisting of a vibrating body.
2   A material medium for transmitting the sound, e.g. air.
3   A device for receiving the sound, i.e. the ear.

From Fig. 2.3 it can be seen that structurally the ear has three parts: the outer ear, the middle ear and the inner ear.

The outer ear

The outer ear comprises a sound receptor, the *auricle* or *pinna* and an inner passage known as the *ear canal* or the *auditory external meatus*. The auricle helps to amplify sound waves in front of the ear. When a hard of hearing person places a hand behind the ear and cups the ear in the direction of the sound he is, in effect, providing an enlargement of the auricle and increased amplification.

The external meatus is a cul-de-sac about the diameter of an ordinary lead pencil and about 25 mm in length. It terminates at

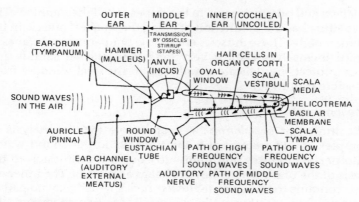

Fig. 2.3 The three parts of the ear

the *ear-drum* or *tympanum* which is a translucent cone-shaped membrane about the same thickness as a sheet of newspaper.

The middle ear

The middle ear is a tiny air-filled cavity approximately 13 mm long by 23 mm high. Although the middle ear is very small, within this space three functions essential to the transmission of sound take place. Firstly, within this space vibrations on the tympanum are carried at increased force to the inner ear by means of a lever system of three bones or *ossicles*. In order of operation, the ossicles are the *malleus*, or *hammer*, which is attached to the tympanum; the *incus* or *anvil*; and the *stapes*, or *stirrup*. The bottom part or footplate of the stapes fits into an aperture in the inner ear termed the *oval window*. To give some idea of the minute size of the ossicles, the stapes, the smallest of the three bones, is only about 3 mm long and weighs scarcely 3 mg.

The second contribution of the middle ear is to maintain an equal air pressure on each side of the tympanum. This pressure is maintained by air which reaches the middle ear through the *eustachian tube*. The eustachian tube opens at its other end into the back of the nose near the adenoids and can be opened by yawning, swallowing or pressing the nostrils together between the finger and thumb and puffing out the cheeks.

Thirdly, the middle ear contains two important muscles: one attached to the tympanum, appropriately called the *tensor tympani* and one connected to the stapes called the *stapedius*. The stapedius has the distinction of being the smallest muscle in the human body. These muscles enable the tympanum and stapes to brace themselves against very loud, low-pitched sounds and thus protect the delicate membrane in the oval window from possible rupture.

The inner ear

The inner ear or *labyrinth* is responsible for the analysis of complex sound frequencies, the transduction of sound waves into nerve impulses and their subsequent transmission to the areas of the brain where they are heard as sounds. The inner ear also contains the three *semi-circular canals* which play no part in hearing, but together with two small, sac-like chambers, the *utricle* and the *saccule*, jointly known as the *vestibule*, they are concerned with the maintenance of balance.

The organ of hearing itself is the *cochlea* – the Greek word for snail – as its external appearance is very similar to the shell of a small snail. If uncoiled, the 2¾ turns of the shell would form a tube about 30-35 mm long and about 5 mm in diameter. Throughout its length the cochlea is divided into two galleries, partly by a bony shelf and partly by a membrane called the *basilar membrane* which varies in thickness from less than 0.001 mm near its basal end to 0.005 mm at the apex of the cochlea. These two galleries are filled with a watery fluid called *perilymph*. The large end of the upper gallery or *scala vestibuli*, connects with the middle ear at the oval window, where the footplate of the stapes makes a fluid-proof seal. The lower gallery, or the *scala tympani*, meets the middle ear at another aperture named the *round window*. The two galleries communicate with each other through a gap termed the *helicotrema*.

From the roof of the upper gallery, another membrane, *Reissner's membrane* (see Fig. 2.4) slopes downwards to form an inner passage shaped like a right-angled triangle, and referred to as the *scala media*. The scala media is also filled with a fluid, *endolymph*. Resting on the part of the basilar membrane that forms the floor of the scala media is the *organ of Corti*, named after Alfrenso Corti who first discovered it in 1851. It is in the organ of Corti that the conversion of sound waves into electrical impulses takes place. Within the organ of Corti are about 23,000 hair cells, arranged in an inner row and four outer rows of rods or

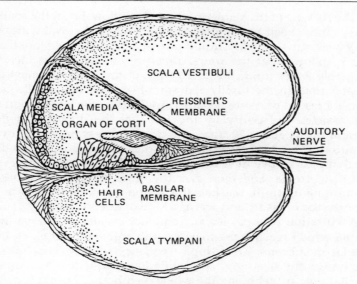

Fig. 2.4 Cross-section of the cochlea

pillars. Near the bases of the hair cells are auditory nerve fibres, between 25,000 and 30,000 in number. Although there is just over one nerve fibre to each hair cell, the relationship is not on a one-to-one basis and a nerve fibre may act like a telephone party-line in supplying endings to many hair cells. The upper ends of the hair cells pass through a thin membrane called the *reticula lamina*, and are embedded in a thicker covering membrane which lies like a flap over the organ of Corti. On leaving the cochlea these fibres twist together, rather like the strands of a rope, to form the auditory nerve which conveys the electrical impulses to the temporal portion of the brain.

How the mechanism works

Sound waves are collected by the auricle and funnelled down the ear canal to the tympanum causing it to vibrate. Middle 'C' on a piano, which is a pure tone, causes the tympanum to make 256 vibrations per second but it is of interest that the ear-drum's vibrations move through a distance equivalent only to the diameter of a hydrogen atom (0.000000001 mm). Vibrations from the tympanum are conducted across the middle ear by the ossicles; they are then transmitted to the cochlea in the inner ear by the rocking of the stapes in the oval window. So far the sound waves have been transmitted through air; at the oval window they pass into fluid. As a liquid provides higher impedance than air, it follows that the sound pressure on the almost incompressible water fluid, the perilymph, of the inner ear must be greater than in the highly compressible air of the middle ear. This increased pressure is partly provided by the lever action of the ossicles and partly by the fact that the diameter of the tympanum is about 20 times the original pressure on the oval window. The action of the stapes on the oval window causes the perilymph to move over Reissner's membrane, round the gap, the helicotrema, and then over the other surface of the basal membrane until it reaches the round window which thus absorbs the pressure and acts as a kind of safety-valve.

A vibration of a particular frequency results in a wave-like ripple which reaches the maximum at a given point along the basilar membrane. Thus, high frequency sounds cause vibrations near the oval window, while low frequency ones cause oscillations further along the whole membrane. The movement of the basilar membrane results in a shearing effect between the hair cells of the organ of Corti and the covering (tectorial) membrane: this, in some way not yet understood, causes an electro-chemical reaction in the nerve fibres. This reaction is transmitted by the auditory nerve which joins with fibres from the semi-circular canals to form the eighth cranial nerve. In the brain the information received is decoded and presented as intelligible sound. It has been estimated that the human ear can identify some 360,000 distinct sounds.

The minuteness of the whole apparatus is impressive. So is its high level of perfection. It has been stated that the ossicles of the middle ear form a mathematically-perfect transmission system, while the contra-actions of the oval and round windows on the perilymph provide an ideal hydraulic system. Finally, the whole process, from the reception of sound waves by the auricle to their interpretation in the auditory cortex of the brain, takes no longer than three-hundredths of a second.

Binaural hearing

This is the term used to describe hearing with two ears; in monaural hearing only one ear is used. Following accident or disease many people have varying degrees of impairment affecting one ear only. Where the 'good' ear is normal or nearly so, they may not be greatly inconvenienced.

There are, however, a number of reasons why two ears are better than one. Experiments have shown that with binaural hearing, sensitivity to sound is increased and, under noisy conditions, speech is more intelligible. Some researchers have also noticed that while the right ear is more efficient at processing speech sounds, the left ear is better with non-speech stimuli such as music. Furthermore, as all stereo enthusiasts know, binaural hearing assists in locating the direction from which a sound comes. Conversely, binaural hearing impairment leads to difficulty in locating sounds. One theory is that binaural hearing helps us to trace the direction of sounds because a sound wave from a given source may strike the ear nearest the sound source fractionally before the other. In a three-dimensional world man's two ears, like his two eyes, work together to locate objects.

Chapter 3

The causes of hearing impairment

An alternative definition of hearing impairment is 'any significant deviation of the normal ear'.[1] In this context the term 'normal ear' refers to the ear of a young adult of between 18 to 22 years of age which has no known defect or history of infection.

Apart from non-organic reasons, such as hysteria, three types of hearing loss may be identified. *Conductive loss* arises through some defect of the outer ear or the middle ear. *Sensorineural loss* arises in the inner ear and beyond. The term 'sensorineural loss' is now preferred to 'perceptive loss', since it emphasises that the impairment may be sensory, arising in the cochlea, or neural, affecting the nerve pathways to the brain. Hearing loss may also be *mixed*, owing to abnormalities affecting both the conductive and the sensorineural mechanisms.

Conductive causes

The main causes of hearing loss due to abnormalities of the sound-conducting mechanism of the ear are as follows:
1 Accidents.
2 Malformations of the outer or middle ear.
3 Obstructions of the outer ear.
4 Infections.
5 Otosclerosis.

Each of the five causes is briefly explained in the following text.

Accidents
These include the rupture of the ear-drum by a blow or explosion

causing sudden pressure in the outer ear. The ear-drum may be perforated by careless syringing or probing.

Malformations

An example of an embryonic malformation is the complete or partial non-formation of the outer ear passage affecting one or both ears. The term *atresia* is used to describe the closure of a normally open body orifice so we may have a congenital atresia of the outer ear passage. In some cases the ear-drum and ossicles are also missing.

Obstructions

The outer ear passage may be blocked by wax or by foreign bodies such as beads inserted by children.

Infections

Otitis externa and *otitis media* are general terms referring respectively to inflammation of the skin lining the outer ear and the middle ear.

Otitis externa is due to bacterial infections and is sometimes called 'swimmer's ear' since it occurs frequently in swimmers who have had water trapped in their ears.

Otitis media is closely related to the eustachian tube. Inflammation may be due to bacteria invading the middle ear through the eustachian tube as a result of head colds, tonsillitis or similar infections of the nose and throat. It may also arise when such infections cause the lining of the eustachian tube to swell or when the tube is obstructed by an enlarged adenoid. In both cases the eustachian tube is unable to fulfil its function of ensuring that the air pressure on the inside of the ear-drum is equal to the atmospheric pressure in the outer ear. In consequence the ear-drum is pushed inwards (retracted). The air remaining in the middle ear is gradually absorbed by the mucous membrane and replaced as fluid. The fluid which accumulates may be non-suppurative, i.e. without pus, or suppurative, i.e. with pus. The retracted drum and the fluid, which impedes this movement of the ossicles, will result in some hearing loss. Acute suppurative otitis media occurs most frequently in children under 7. It is accompanied by severe pain; the drum may be pushed outwards (distended) by the pressure of the pus and, if not treated by antibiotics or released by the otologist, will cause the ear drum to rupture or perforate, after which the pain will subside. A danger of suppurative otitis media is that the infection will spread to the air cells of the mastoid process causing mastoiditis.

Both non-suppurative and suppurative otitis media may become chronic conditions. An example of the former is *adhesive otitis media* in which poor ventilation by the eustachian tube may cause fluid to accumulate insidiously in the middle ear. In some cases an inflammatory condition may be neutralised by antibiotics but the fluid, now sterile, remains in the inner ear and, if untreated, becomes thick and gluey. Adhesions may further impede the movement of the ossicles so that the transmission of sound to the inner ear is reduced. Calcium deposits can lead to a thickening of the ear-drum resulting in tympanosclerosis.

Chronic suppurative otitis media may be either 'safe' or 'dangerous'. In the 'safe' condition the discharge through the perforated ear-drum is clear and odourless and the hearing loss relatively slight. The 'dangerous' type of infection is evidenced by a bloody, evil-smelling discharge which may indicate a cholesteatoma or pseudotumour. A cholesteatoma contains bone-destroying matter which may destroy the ossicles. If allowed to spread to the inner ear, a treatable, conductive impairment will change into an irreversible, sensorineural loss and can represent a threat to life.

Otosclerosis

Ballantyne[2] points out that the term otosclerosis, meaning a hardening of the ear bone, is a misnomer since the condition is characterised by a local replacement of the normal, hard, mature bone with a soft, spongy, immature bone, usually over the footplate of the stapes which becomes fixed in the oval window, thus impeding the transmission of vibrations to the fluid of the inner ear. Initially otosclerosis may be unilateral but later both ears may be affected. Otosclerosis is a progressive condition and may ultimately involve the cochlea resulting in a mixed impairment. The term 'pathological enigma' has been applied to otosclerosis since there are still no firm conclusions regarding the causes. It has, however, some interesting characteristics:

1   Otosclerosis is the commonest cause of hearing impairment from adulthood to middle age; most cases are reported around the age of 30.

2 The condition is estimated to be twice as common in women than in men. Hearing loss is often associated with pregnancy or the menopause.

3 It is more prevalent in white than in black races, and among the fair-haired.

4 There is usually, though not always, a family history of 'deafness'.

5 People with otosclerosis claim to hear better in a noise. This symptom is known as the *paracusis of Willis* after the otologist by whom it was first reported.

Sensorineural causes

The causes of sensorineural hearing impairment are varied and complex. They can be most conveniently classified according to the time at which the impairment took place rather than into the two simple categories of congenital and acquired loss. A useful classification is into pre-natal, paranatal and post-natal causes, according to whether the loss occurred before, during or after birth respectively:

1 Pre-natal causes:
   (a) Genetic or familial hearing loss;
   (b) Viral infections.

2 Paranatal causes:
   (a) Anoxia;
   (b) Kernicterus;
   (c) Prematurity;
   (d) Injury.

3 Post-natal causes:
   (a) Viral or bacterial infections;
   (b) Toxic antibodies;
   (c) Noise-induced hearing loss;
   (d) Accidents;
   (e) Presbyacusis.

Pre-natal causes

Genetic or familial hearing loss. It is useful to distinguish hereditary deafness from congenital deafness. The latter category implies that the hearing loss was present at birth and may include acquired as well as hereditary factors. Hereditary loss applies to those cases where the causes were present in the fertilised ovum and transmitted as a dominant or recessive characteristic. Where one parent carries a dominant deaf gene the risk of a hearing impaired baby is as high as 50 per cent. In the recessive form in which both parents must be carriers of a hearing characteristic that produces sensorineural impairment, the risk is only 25 per cent.

Viral infections. Hearing loss is the most common of all abnormalities, which may be multiple, arising from maternal rubella. The risk to hearing is highest in the first 12–16 weeks of pregnancy when the ear is developing. The birth of babies handicapped by congenital rubella can be prevented by vaccination. The DHSS has set a target for the rubella vaccination of 95 per cent of all girls aged between 11 and 13 in each health authority. Health authorities are also encouraged to ensure that serological screening for immunity to rubella followed by vaccination, where appropriate, is available to all women of childbearing age who have not been vaccinated at school. All antenatal patients should also be screened for rubella so as to identify those who will need vaccination after the birth of their babies.[3] Other viral infections include syphilis and maternal influenza.

Paranatal causes

These arise from the hazards of birth.

Anoxia (shortage of oxygen). This can occur in a baby as a result of a difficult birth. It is believed to result in some cases in hearing loss although the reason is not clear.

Kernicterus (nuclear jaundice) results when a mother lacking the Rhesus factor (antigen) conceives a Rhesus positive baby. To combat the Rhesus factor the mother's body produces antibodies. In a first pregnancy the antibody count is low and the baby is not at risk. By the third pregnancy, however, the antibody concentration is sufficient to destroy the baby's red blood cells and release a bile pigment (bilirubin) into the child's bloodstream. Before birth the bilirubin is detoxicated by the mother's liver. After birth, however, the baby's immature liver cannot cope and the concentration of bilirubin in its bloodstream rises causing jaundice. If within a few hours of birth the blood is not entirely replaced, bilirubin may become deposited in the cochlea causing a sensorineural loss.

Prematurity sometimes results in sensorineural loss probably because the immature liver contributes to the development of kernicterus. Prematurity relates not to the length of pregnancy but weight at birth; a baby with a birth weight less than 2.5 kg (5.5 lb) is, conventionally, immature.

Injury to the brain and cochlea may occasionally be due to the use of instruments during delivery.

Post-natal causes

These may arise at any time after birth.

Virus or bacterial infections, the most common of which are mumps and measles (rubeola), may cause unilateral or bilateral hearing loss. Bacterial meningitis, either meningococcal or tubercular damaging the cochlea or auditory nerve can cause severe or total loss of hearing which sometimes occurs several months after the onset of the meningitis.

Toxic antibodies such as streptomycin, neomycin and kanamycin have been found to have side-effects producing mild to profound hearing loss.

Noise-induced hearing loss may be due to either sudden or continuous exposure to sound. The potential damage to hearing by a given noise therefore depends both on its intensity and duration. Sudden exposure to high intensity noise over 150 decibels (dB) will cause extensive damage, usually bilateral, to the drums and ossicles. The cochlea may escape if disruption of the ossicles prevents the full intensity of the noise being transmitted to the perilymph fluid. Continuous exposure to high intensity noise, as occurs in some industrial occupations, is associated with damage to the sensitive hair cells of the cochlea.

Accidents involving head injuries may damage the cochlea. Middle ear surgery is not without risk. The incidence of cochlea hearing loss from stapedectomy, for example, is variously estimated at from 1 per cent to 5 per cent of operated cases.

Presbyacusis, or hearing loss associated with old age, is caused by independent, degenerative changes in the auditory neural pathways and in the cochlea, resulting in reduced sensitivity to high frequency sounds. Although reduction in auditory sensitivity commences in adolescence, hearing difficulties only become noticeable around the early and late 60s for men and women respectively. 'Recruitment', described below, is a feature of presbyacusis. Presbyacusis may be related to and accentuate hearing loss from other causes such as occupational exposure to noise.

Recognising the type of hearing loss

Whether a particular case of hearing impairment is conductive, sensorineural or mixed can only be reliably determined by an otologist after a detailed examination including audiometry. A rough assessment of whether an individual has a predominantly conductive or sensorineural loss can be made from the signs tabulated in Table 3.1.

Table 3.1 Characteristics of different types of hearing loss

	Conductive loss	Sensorineural loss
Typical speech	Low and soft, as the person can hear his or her own voice through bone conduction	Speech is loud with a tendency to shout, as the person had difficulty in hearing his own voice
Toleration of loudness	Loud sounds and speech can be tolerated	Loud sounds and speech of an intensity considerably above the threshold of hearing may cause discomfort due to *recruitment* or an exaggerated sensation of hearing following a slight increase in the intensity of sound
Background noise	Hearing is better in a noise	Noise may adversely affect discrimination due to recruitment

References

1   Newby. *Audiology*, 4th edn, 1979, p.61.
2   Ballantyne, J. *Deafness*, 2nd edn, Ch. 13, p.109., J. and A. Churchill.
3   See DHSS Circulars, HC(79)14, June 1979, and DA(80)15 8, August 1980.

Chapter 4

The ascertainment, diagnosis and measurement of hearing impairment

Ascertainment, diagnosis and measurement of hearing loss are the essential first steps in auditory rehabilitation.

Ascertainment

Both children and adults may have an undetected hearing loss until the impairment is revealed by screening. Screening is not concerned with the cause, type or severity of hearing loss but only the detection of those who are irresponsive to certain sound stimuli within normal limits. The importance of screening, the methods used and the agencies involved differ according to whether the subject is a pre-school child, a pupil at school or an adult.

The pre-school child

Since the development of speech and language depend on hearing, delay in ascertaining a pre-lingual auditory impairment can have far-reaching consequences for the subsequent intellectual, emotional and social development of the child concerned. Considerable research has been undertaken into the screening of new-born babies for hearing loss by noting neurological and physiological responses to sound stimulation. In Brain Stem Electric Response Audiometry, electrodes placed on the forehead, scalp and mastoid bone sense electric signals generated by the auditory nerve when stimulated by sound. Other physiological responses to sound, such as breathing, heartbeats or head or eye movements can be noted for screening

25

purposes. At the time of writing, a fully automatic micro-processor-controlled newborn hearing device known as an Auditory Response Cradle is being widely tested.[1] Such devices do not, however, obviate the need for further screening, which should be undertaken at about the age of 7 months. Before this age, babies are generally unable to sit unsupported and their responses to sound are unreliable. In 1981 a report of the DHSS Advisory Committee on Services for Hearing Impaired People[2] endorsed earlier recommendations[3] that screening for hearing should take place at 7–8 months, 2½–3 years, on school entry and during the later primary school period at about 8–9 years. The duties of local authorities with regard to assessment are stated in Chapter 7.

Taylor[4] has stated that 'the application of screening tests is not universal and the standards of practice are not universally good.' For cost-effective reasons some authorities only screen babies who, for such reasons as a family history of deafness, appear on 'high risk' registers even though only about 50 per cent of hearing impaired babies appear on such lists[3]. Taylor further suggests that:

The medical and allied professions do not take sufficient notice of the opinion of the mother about the state of her baby's hearing. I have found that if a mother says her new baby is deaf, she is invariably right. It is for this reason that I would recommend that we not only screen all babies between the ages of seven and nine months for hearing but we supplement this by a simple questioning of the mother, asking her if she has any reason to doubt the normality of her baby's hearing. If either of these procedures indicate a doubt, then I would recommend that the baby is examined without further delay by a doctor experienced in the test procedures appropriate to babies.

The DHSS Advisory Committee recommended that because of her knowledge and participation in the physical and mental development of the young child and her relationship with mothers, the most suitable person to undertake screening for hearing impairment of children under 5 years is the health visitor. A statutory duty is laid on health authorities to ensure that a mother is visited by a health visitor after the birth of her baby. Screening procedures are simple and involve the use of distraction, performance and speech discrimination tests.

Distraction or localisation tests

These are used at about 7–8 months aim to ensure that the baby can hear and locate quick sounds of about 35 dB. The test should be conducted by two trained personnel known as the 'tester' and the 'distractor'. The distractor will gain the baby's interest with a suitable toy and then 'plateau' the child's attention by ceasing the play activity or hiding the toy. The tester, who will be located behind and out of sight of the baby at a standard distance and angle of 3ft and 45° from the test ear respectively, will immediately present the sound signal at ear-level. Initially the tester may check response to normal environmental sounds by gently stroking a spoon round the inside rim of a cup. This procedure, however, covers too wide a spectrum of frequencies to be used as a test item, and it is necessary to test the response to both low and high frequency sounds, the former by the use of low frequency voice sounds (e.g. a repeated 'Boo-oo-oo-oo'), the latter by a high-pitched rattle and 's-s-s-s-' sounds. Sounds should be varied from left to right, or the baby will anticipate their direction. Distraction testing can be done at home or at the clinic but it is essential that ambient noise does not exceed 30 dB and that both the tester and distractor have normal hearing.

Performance tests

These, used with speech tests (both are necessary) at 2½–3 years, aim to provide information of the minimal loudness level at which speech is audible to the child. After initial conditioning, in which the child is taught to make a clear response to a stimulus, the child is given both low and high frequency sound signals to perform a given action, e.g. adding a brick to a tower. The low frequency signal may be a simple word, e.g. 'go'; the high frequency an 's' sound e.g. 'Sammy Snake says hiss.' The tester should gradually reduce the intensity of speech and test both ears by moving gradually to above 3–4ft each side of the child. For both low and high frequency sounds, three satisfactory responses should be required.

Speech discrimination tests

These require a child to identify toys or pictures, each selected because they have easily comprehended monosyllabic names, or to point to parts of the body or objects in the room. The instructions are given from behind or at each side of the child, initially at normal conversational level and then at reduced intensities.

A child failing an initial screening test should be retested after a short interval normally of from 1–4 weeks. Between 1–2 per cent of babies tested fail two screening tests.

The school child

Research findings show that while children with profound hearing loss are usually detected early, those with a less severe impairment are discovered much later. As stated earlier, the DHSS recommends that children other than those at high risk or with other special circumstances should be routinely tested twice during school life. From age 3 years onwards, performance testing may be superseded by the pure-tone audiometric testing used for adults described later in this chapter. Such testing may be on a group or individual basis. Group procedures enable several children to be screened simultaneously with a consequent saving in time. Anderson,[5] however, estimates that possibly 40 per cent of those tested may fail their first group hearing test; hearing impairment is found in only 5–12 per cent of subjects retested. In doubtful cases, initial group testing by the school nurse, physiological measurement technician (audiology) or peripatetic teacher of the deaf is followed by individual screening and testing by an audiologist. Teachers have an important role in detecting hearing loss. Slowness or persistent inattention should arouse the suspicion that the pupil is experiencing hearing difficulties. Such cases will be referred to the school doctor.

Adults

Most hearing loss in adult life is insidious in onset and progressive in severity and the subject may be unaware of any impairment until this is discovered inadvertently at a medical examination or by industrial screening. The International Labour Office recommends[6] that a worker to be continuously exposed to a noise level exceeding 85 dB should be medically examined before employment followed by periodical examinations at intervals depending on the magnitude of the exposure hazard. Such examinations should include a clinical examination of the ears and a screening (or simplified) audiometric test. All audiograms should be preserved by the employer.

In other cases increasing communication difficulties at home and work will cause a person to seek help.

Diagnosis

Diagnosis has been defined as detective work with logic as its basis. The key figure in the diagnosis of hearing impairment, and within the National Health Service, the person to whom all concerned with rehabilitation are ultimately responsible, is the ear, nose and throat consultant or otologist. Children identified by screening should be routinely referred to an otologist although this may not take place. As the DHSS Advisory Committee observed:[2]

There is no national pattern of referral after a child has failed the screening test for hearing. Sometimes the child will be referred to his family doctor, who will decide whether to take any further action. In other areas, the community health services may have an arrangement with the GP for the child to be referred direct to the community clinic for further tests. Whatever procedures are followed, we are concerned that there is often far too long an interval between the time when suspicion of a hearing impairment is aroused and the subsequent follow up action.

The Committee recommended that clinical medical officers with special training in audiology should undertake sessions in community clinics to which children referred from screening programmes should be sent. Children requiring more specialist advice would be referred to special Hearing Assessment Centres which would be the focal point of the basic service.

Adults with hearing loss or other ear trouble will be sent to their general practitioner. Not all GPs are sympathetic to hearing loss and a patient may need to insist on seeing a consultant. It is important to recognise that developments in middle ear surgery and hearing aid technology may enable statements made by consultants many years ago that 'nothing could be done' now to be revised. An examination by an otologist must precede the issue of an NHS hearing aid.

Information provided by or on behalf of a patient is important in assisting the otologist with his diagnosis. Clear answers should therefore be prepared to such questions as the following:

1 When was the hearing loss first noticed?
2 What events, if any, are associated with the loss – e.g. an

accident, colds, noise, pregnancy etc?
3   Is there any family history of 'deafness'?
4   What illnesses has the patient had since birth?
5   What symptoms are present additional to hearing loss, e.g.
    head noises, vertigo, discharge, pain?
6   Does hearing seem better in noisy surroundings?
7   Are loud noises or speech uncomfortable?

The otologist will also observe the patient's general de-
meanour and attitude to hearing loss as well as whether he
speaks loudly or softly, presents one ear to the speaker or
attempts to speech-read.

In the physical examination of the patient's ears, nose and
throat, attention will be given to the colour and texture of the
ear-drums and whether these are perforated, retracted or bulge
outwards. The patency of the eustachian tube will be tested and
any abnormalities, such as enlarged adenoids that prevent their
proper functioning, observed.

The aim of diagnostic testing is to obtain precise information
regarding the severity and site of the hearing impairment. Prior
to the introduction of audiometers and other diagnostic aids,
otologists relied on tuning forks to compare hearing by air and
bone conduction. In one such test (Rinne) a vibrating tuning fork
is first held at the auricle and, when no longer heard by the
patient, transferred to the mastoid process. A 'negative Rinne',
in which the tone is louder at the mastoid, indicates a conductive
loss located in either the outer or middle ear. A 'positive Rinne',
in which the tone is louder at the auricle, is characteristic either
of normal hearing or a sensorineural loss. Another popular test
(Weber) shows whether a unilateral loss is conductive or
sensorineural by placing a vibrating tuning fork on the middle of
the patient's forehead. With normal hearing the tone is heard
equally in both ears. A louder tone in the worst ear indicates a
conductive loss; a sensorineural loss is typified by a louder tone
in the better ear.

While these simple but ingenious tests are still used, the
otologist is now assisted in his diagnosis, prognosis and
management of hearing impairment by a battery of tests that the
audiologist has at his disposal. Simple pure-tone and speech
audiometry are described later in this chapter. Other procedures
are outside the scope of a non-specialist book. Impedance testing
involving tympanometry, intra-aural muscle reflex testing and

eustachian tube evaluation provides information on the normality or otherwise of the middle ear. Evoked response audiometry applications such as electrocochleography can indicate the potential of the cochlea and auditory nerve and identify the 'sensory' and 'neural' elements in sensorineural loss.

Measurement

Pure-tone and speech audiometry are important not only for diagnostic purposes but also in evaluating the extent to which a person is handicapped or disabled by hearing loss and the rehabilitative help that can be given. An understanding of pure-tone and speech audiometry requires some knowledge of decibels and audiometers.

Decibels

Sound is measured in decibels. A decibel is not a unit such as a mile or a metre but a *ratio*. The sound produced by two bees is twice that of one bee. Similarly the noise of two similar racing cars is double that of one car. Although the cars will make vastly more noise than the bees, the relative increase in sound will be the same in both cases.

All measurements must start somewhere. If we wish to measure the temperature (using the Centigrade scale) the reference is the freezing-point of water. Temperatures lower than that at which water freezes are described as 'below zero'. The zero or reference for the decibel is called the threshold of hearing which may be considered as the quietest pure tone audible at a given frequency to a person with normal hearing. In a simplified form, therefore, a decibel can be expressed as either:

$$\frac{\text{Sound intensity}}{\text{Reference sound intensity}} \quad \text{or} \quad \frac{\text{Sound pressure}}{\text{Reference sound pressure}}$$

Decibels measure both sound intensity and sound pressure. Intensity is the energy given out by a sound-source, e.g. a hi-fi speaker. Pressure is the force exerted on a resisting surface, e.g. the ear-drum. Intensity and pressure, although having different reference points, are related since sound energy increases as the square of sound pressure. Thus, as shown in Table 4.1, a tenfold increase in pressure corresponds to a hundredfold (10 × 10) increase in sound energy.

Table 4.1 Sound intensity and sound pressure units and their decibel equivalents

Sound intensity ratio	Decibel equivalent	Sound pressure ratio
1:1	0	1:1
100:1	10	10:1 (10^1)
10,000:1	20	100:1 (10^2)
1,000,000:1	30	1,000:1 (10^3)
1,000,000,000:1	40	10,000:1 (10^4)
10,000,000,000:1	50	100,000:1 (10^5)
1,000,000,000,000:1	60	1,000,000:1 (10^6)
100,000,000,000,000:1	70	10,000,000:1 (10^7)

Since the smallest audible sound is about one ten-millionth of the loudest sound the ear can tolerate, we need to reduce this range to manageable size. Any number can be expressed in terms of 10 to a given power, i.e. 1,000 is 10 × 10 × 10 or 10^3. Originally sound was measured in Bels named after Alexander Graham Bell. One Bel equalled a tenfold increase in sound energy. Similarly three Bels corresponded to 10^3. The awkward number of 1,000,000,000,000 could therefore be reduced to 12 Bels or 12 tenfold increases. The Bel, however, was too imprecise for electronic engineers and in 1929 the decibel or one-tenth of a Bel was adopted.

Most audiometric applications are concerned with sound pressure. How the 10 million range in sound pressure is compressed into a spectrum of 140 dB is shown by Fig. 4.1, which also relates some everyday sound to decibels.

Audiometers

Audiometers may be manual or automatic. With the former, the operator is engaged throughout the test in selecting frequency and intensity levels, presenting the signal tones to each ear and manually recording the subject's responses on an audiogram. Automatic audiometers only require the operator to instruct the subject, exchange the audiogram chart and return the audiogram table to the start position after the test. A Bekesey automatic audiometer is programmed to present a predetermined set of frequencies to each ear, the subject recording his own threshold levels by pressing a button immediately the tone is heard. The button is released when the signal is inaudible. The results are

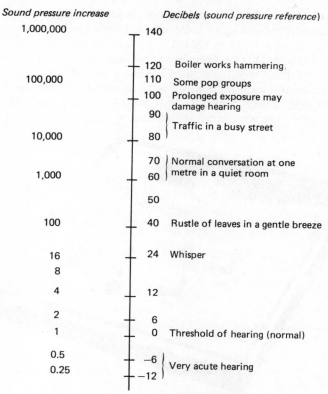

Fig. 4.1 Intensities of common sounds in decibels

automatically recorded. Computerised audiometers, claimed to be more reliable, and faster to operate than other manual or automatic instruments, are being developed.

Audiometers may also be categorised as 'screening' or 'diagnostic'. A screening audiometer (Fig. 4.2), as used for pure-tone testing by air conduction in schools or factories, is a simple instrument with controls limited to selectors for frequencies and hearing level. The frequency-level selector tests hearing at frequencies of 250, 500, 750, 1,000, 1,500, 2,000, 3,000, 4,000, 6,000, and 8,000 Hz. The hearing-level selector presents each frequency at a defined sound pressure range from 0–80 dB.

Apart from the earphone the essential features of a simple, manually operated, diagnostic audiometer for clinical use are shown in Fig. 4.2. The instrument illustrated can, by pure-tone audiometry, establish air conduction thresholds in 5 dB steps over a range from −10 dB to 120 dB (with +20 dB) at nine frequencies from 250 to 8,000 Hz. Thresholds for bone conduction from −10 dB to 60 dB at seven frequencies from 250 to 4,000 Hz can be determined, enabling hearing to be tested at frequencies of 250, 500, 1,000, 1,500, 2,000, 3,000, 4,000, 6,000 and 8,000 Hz. The instrument shown cannot be used for speech audiometry.

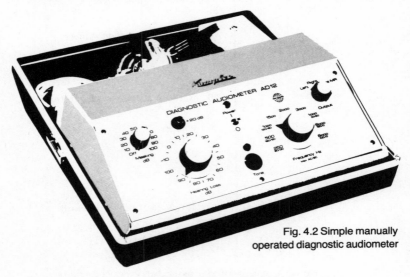

Fig. 4.2 Simple manually
operated diagnostic audiometer

Other features of a diagnostic audiometer may include a masking device and facilities for speech audiometry, such as a VU (volume units) meter which enables the loudness of speech input to be monitored. The function of the masking device is to obviate cross-hearing. In tests of bone conduction and also of air conduction, where the acuity of the two ears differs by more than 40 dB, tests may be distorted because test sounds presented to the worst ear may be heard in the better ear. This distortion affects accurate diagnosis where it is essential to know the difference in bone and air conduction for each ear. Masking ensures that the better ear does not hear the test signal by presenting it with a 'white noise' or other masking sound. (White noise is continuous noise, e.g. the hissing of steam, in which high, middle and low frequencies are equally presented.)

Modern audiometers are calibrated to the standard adopted by the International Standards Organisation. This standard set 0 dB as the threshold of hearing for pure-tone audiometers and was based on a survey of the hearing of a large number of otologically-normal people aged 18–30 years. An 'otologically-normal subject' was defined as 'a person in a normal state of health who is free from all signs or symptoms of ear disease and from wax in the ear canal and has no history of undue exposure to noise'.

Applications of audiometry

An audiometric examination for diagnostic purposes comprises a battery of tests. Pure-tone testing by air and bone conduction and speech reception tests may be complemented by procedures such as impedance testing of the ear-drum and the stapedius muscle of the middle ear. Other, so-called 'site of lesion' tests, designed to indicate the precise area in the auditory system producing symptoms of abnormal auditory function, include procedures to determine recruitment and tone decay. Readers wishing to know more about audiometry other than pure-tone and speech testing, should refer to one of the many excellent textbooks on audiology.

Pure-tone audiometry

The purpose of pure-tone audiometry is to determine the threshold of hearing for air and bone conduction at selected frequencies.

For air conduction testing, a pure-tone signal will be presented to each ear through a headphone. The operator will usually begin by presenting an initial test tone of 1,000 Hz to the better ear at, say, 40 dB. The subject will indicate that the tone has been heard by raising a finger or pressing a button. Following each positive response the intensity of the test tone is reduced in 10 dB steps until the subject fails to acknowledge the signal. The tone is then raised 5 dB. If heard, the tone is reduced 10 dB; if not, it is raised in 5 dB steps until it is acknowledged. Thus, in what is known as the 'up 5–down 10' method, an increment of 5 dB is used if the preceding tone was not heard and a 10 dB reduction when the tone has been received. After the threshold for 1,000 Hz has been determined in the better ear, the procedure is repeated at frequencies of 2,000, 4,000, 8,000, 500 and 250 Hz in that order. If between each octave (an octave is the pitch interval between two tones, one of which is twice the frequency of the other) the thresholds show a significant rise or fall, testing may be done for the half octaves 750, 1,500, 3,000 and 6,000 Hz to obtain a better assessment of the overall hearing configuration. Testing of the second ear usually begins not at 1,000 Hz but with the last frequency used to test the opposite ear.

For bone conduction testing a vibrator will usually be applied in turn to the mastoid of each ear, although some authorities prefer the frontal bone rather than the mastoid. With bone conduction a masking sound is usually presented to the ear not under test.

It is important to remember that a pure-tone audiogram gives little indication of the everyday consequences of hearing impairment.

Speech audiometry

In speech audiometry, word or sentence tests, either on tape or by the live voice, are presented in turn to each ear by a headphone. Alternatively, free-field testing, in which the words are delivered to both ears at a measured level of loudness by amplifier or voice, may be used. Free-field testing helps in estimating the likely benefit in normal circumstances from a hearing aid. Apart from hearing aid prescription and other rehabilitation procedures such as speech-reading and auditory training, speech audiometry is useful in diagnosis and predicting the probable results of middle ear surgery. The results of testing are charted on a speech audiogram.

Some useful results provided by speech audiometry are the SRT or Speech Reception Threshold; the PB or Speech Discrimination Score; the MCL or Most Comfortable Loudness Level and the TD or Threshold of Discomfort.

The SRT is the lowest decibel level at which 50 per cent of a list of monosyllabic or spondee words can be identified. (A spondee is a word of two syllables in which equal stress is laid on each syllable e.g. 'mush room', 'sun set'.) This threshold approximates closely to the average dB for frequencies of 500, 1,000 and 2,000 Hz. The normal SRT is 10 to 20 dB above the average pure-tone threshold at 500, 1,000 and 2,000 Hz.

PB tests are so called because they test ability to discriminate between the 16 vowel and 22 consonant sounds to be found in

English by using a list of 50 phonetically-balanced (PB), one-syllable words, e.g. 'saw', 'book', 'two', at various dB levels above the SRT. Vowel sounds are easier to hear because they are lower in frequency and higher in intensity than consonants. The difference between the lowest vowel sound *aw* and the softest consonant sound *th* is almost 30 dB. The score is plotted as a percentage of correct response. A general guide for the evaluation of word discrimination scores is shown in Table 4.2.

Table 4.2 Evaluation of word discrimination scores in PB tests

Score	Evaluation
90–100%	Normal limits
75–90%	Slight difficulty comparable to listening over a telephone
60–75%	Moderate difficulty
50–60%	Poor discrimination, difficulty in following conversation
Below 50%	Very poor discrimination, difficulty in following running speech

PB tests can be used to distinguish between conductive and sensorineural loss. A score below the normal limits is generally an indication of sensorineural involvement.

The MCL is the loudness level at which the test material (spondee words) or cold, running speech e.g. a rapidly-delivered lecture at a monotonous level without peaks, is understood. The MCL indicates for each ear, or, when free-field testing is used, both ears together, the number of dB above his SRT at which the subject can most comfortably hear speech. For people with normal hearing this will be about 40 dB above their SRT. With sensorineural impairment, where recruitment is present, however, the MCL may be only 10 dB above the SRT and an increase of 15–20 dB above the SRT may cause discomfort. This is clearly of importance when prescribing a hearing aid.

The TD or *Threshold of Discomfort* is the sound pressure level at which speech becomes uncomfortably loud. By subtracting the SRT from the TD we have the *dynamic range* which indicates the range of useful hearing in each ear or for both ears with free-field testing.

Audiometric evaluation

Audiometric evaluation together with an examination by a consultant otologist are the essential first steps in any programme for the rehabilitation of hearing impaired persons. For rehabilitation purposes it is necessary to equate the quantitative measurement of hearing loss shown by a pure-tone audiogram to a given degree of handicap or disability.

A classification of hearing handicap based on the performance of the ear at the three speech frequencies of 500, 1,000 and 2,000 Hz, and formulated by the American Academy of Ophthalmology and Otolaryngology, is shown in Fig. 4.3. A second classification by S. R. Mawson, a British otologist, is reproduced, with permission, in Fig. 4.4.

Hearing threshold level	Class	Degree of handicap	Average hearing threshold level for 500, 1,000 and 2,000 Hz in better ear		Ability to understand speech
			More than	Not more than	
25 dB	A	Not significant		25 dB	No significant difficulty with faint speech
40 dB	B	Slight handicap	25 dB	40 dB	Difficulty only with faint speech
55 dB	C	Mild handicap	40 dB	55 dB	Frequent difficulty with normal speech
70 dB	D	Marked handicap	55 dB	70 dB	Frequent difficulty with loud speech
90 dB	E	Severe handicap	70 dB	90 dB	Can understand only shouted or amplified speech
90 dB +	F	Extreme handicap	90 dB		Usually cannot understand even amplified speech

Fig. 4.3 Classes of hearing handicap

In evaluating disability and handicap, however, many other factors will have to be given consideration besides the information given by pure-tone and speech audiograms. These will be considered later in this book. An audiogram is, in fact, no more than a measurement of the hearing loss of a given person at a given time.

Classification	Social difficulty	Clinic voice test	Pure-tone audiograms
Normal hearing	None	18 ft or more	No loss over 10 dB
Slight deafness	Long-distance speech	Not over 12 ft	10–30 dB loss
Moderate deafness	Short-distance speech	Not over 3 ft	Up to 60 dB loss
Severe deafness	All unamplified voices	Raised voice at meatus	Over 60 dB loss
Total deafness	Voices never heard	Nil	Over 90 dB loss

Fig. 4.4 Clinical classifications of deafness

Interpreting audiograms

The interpretation of audiograms is the province of the otologist and the clinical audiologist. It is dangerous for the layman to attempt such interpretation, for two reasons. First, an audiogram configuration may be due to more than one cause; secondly, it is necessary to consider the pure-tone audiogram in association with the patient's case history, physical signs and symptoms observed by the otologist from the examination of the patient's ears, nose and throat and supplementary information obtained where necessary from speech and impedance and other differential diagnostic audiometric tests. It is useful, however, to understand in broad outline the principal facts to remember when looking at pure-tone and speech audiograms.

Pure-tone audiograms

In a pure-tone audiogram frequencies are shown along the horizontal axis and intensities on the vertical axis. The hearing threshold by air and bone conduction at each frequency is separately plotted for each ear at co-ordinated points. A typical coding for unmasked and masked testing is as follows:

| Ear | Unmasked | | Masked | |
	Air Conduction (AC)	Bone Conduction (BC)	AC	BC
Left	X	< or]	□	◄
Right	O	> or [	△	►

A pure-tone audiogram can be divided into zones for lower (125–250 Hz), middle (500, 1,000, 2,000 Hz) and higher frequency areas (4,000–8,000 Hz). This zoning enables a hearing loss to be described as affecting the low, middle, or high frequency range or any combination of these.

Comparison of the pure-tone hearing thresholds for air and bone conduction indicate whether hearing loss is conductive, sensorineural or mixed:

1 A conductive loss is shown by normal bone conduction and depressed air conduction thresholds.
2 A sensorineural loss is indicated when both air and bone conduction thresholds are reduced by approximately the same amount so that the configurations tend to intertwine.
3 A mixed loss is characterised when both bone and air conduction thresholds are depressed with the air conduction curve more severely affected.
4 The conductive element in hearing loss lies between the bone conduction and air conduction curves. This bone-air gap is considered significant when it exceeds 15–20 dB.
5 The sensorineural element in hearing loss is the portion between the zero line of a pure-tone audiogram and the bone conduction curve. Where the zero and bone conduction lines coincide there is no sensorineural loss.
6 The overall loss due to both conductive and sensorineural causes is the distance between the zero line and the air conduction curve.

Where the audiometric pattern is relatively flat and regular the effect of pure-tone sensitivity on speech reception can be estimated by averaging the air condition thresholds at 500, 1,000 and 2,000 Hz for each ear. The estimated SRT is the result of such averaging. Where the air conduction threshold at one of the three frequencies differs by more than 20 dB from the other two it is usual to base the estimated SRT on the average of the best two threshold levels.

Certain pure-tone configurations are associated with specific pathological conditions. To give two examples:

1 In pure otosclerosis where there is no cochlear involvement, the bone conduction threshold is depressed at frequencies of 500, 1,000, 2,000 and 4,000 Hz with the greatest depression at 2,000 Hz. This phenomenon is known as the *Carhart notch*. This is further explained below.

2   Sensorineural loss due to prolonged exposure to high intensity noise affects air and bone curves equally and is evidenced by an audiogram in which auditory sensitivity is progressively worse between 3,000 and 6,000 Hz. With continuous exposure the loss spreads to the lower frequencies.

Speech audiograms

The measures obtained from speech audiometry have been described earlier in this chapter (p. 37). Speech audiograms show intensities on the horizontal axis and speech discrimination scores as a percentage of words presented by the client on the vertical axis.

A speech audiogram shows the extent to which the client's ability to discriminate speech improves when the intensity is raised above the normal speech reception threshold. Discrimination scores at a given frequency are plotted to the right of the zero line or normal SRT.

Speech discrimination curves are useful in determining the type of hearing loss and the benefit to be derived from a hearing aid:

1   With a pure conductive loss the discrimination curve will be parallel to that for a person with normal hearing but further to the right. Thus amplification by means of a hearing aid will enable the person with a pure conductive impairment to hear speech normally.

2   In an ear with a severe conductive loss a reduction in speech discrimination suggests a sensorineural element.

3   A parabolic curve in which the PB score reduces or 'rolls over' after a certain intensity level is associated with factors such as distortion and recruitment which limit the ability of the ear to handle speech signals delivered at a high level of intensity.

Examples of audiograms

Some common audiometric configurations are shown in Figs. 4.5–4.9. Figure 4.5 is the pure-tone, pre-operative audiogram for the right ear of a patient with a conductive loss due to otosclerosis. The bone conduction curve shows the characteristic Carhart notch pattern. Carhart, an American otologist, reported in 1951 that prior to surgery (at that time the fenestration operation) the bone conduction of persons with otosclerosis could not be measured accurately because of an inner ear block caused by the fixed stapes impeding the movement of the inner ear fluids. On average this impedance resulted in a lowering of the bone conduction thresholds of 5 dB at 500 Hz, 10 dB at 1,000 Hz, 15 dB at 2,000 Hz and 20 dB at 4,000 Hz. In Fig. 4.5 this notching is pronounced at 2,000 Hz.

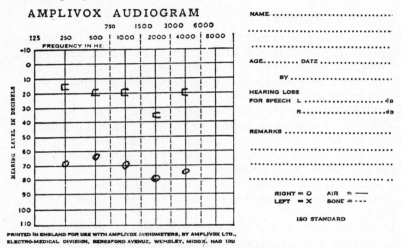

Fig. 4.5 Pre-operative pure-tone audiogram showing significant bone-air gap and Carhart notch

The difference between the bone and air conduction thresholds is the 'bone-air' gap. The aim of middle ear surgery for the restoration of hearing is the reduction or elimination of this gap. Figure 4.6, which is the audiogram after stapedectomy of the same patient as in Fig. 4.5, shows that this aim has been successfully achieved. It will be noticed that the Carhart notch has disappeared since it resulted from the otosclerotic condition and not from sensorineural causes. By averaging the losses on the pre-operative audiogram at frequencies of 500, 1,000 and 2,000 Hz, i.e. $65 + 70 + 80 = 215 \div 3 = 72$ we can estimate that the speech threshold in this case would be about 72 dB.

Figure 4.7 is the speech audiogram of another case of otosclerosis. The speech discrimination curve for a person with normal hearing is shown for comparison on the left. It will be seen that the speech discrimination score or PB curve is very similar to that for normal hearing except that it is necessary to elevate the intensity level by the amount of hearing loss. In this

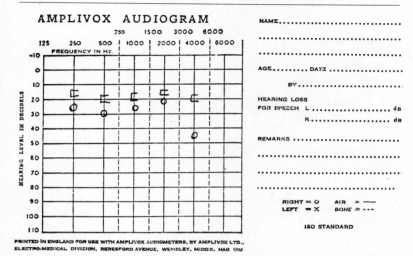

Fig. 4.6 Post-operative pure-tone audiogram showing reduction of bone-air gap

case the intensity level had to be raised to 60 dB before a 100 per cent score was obtained. Persons with this type of pure conductive loss are ideal-candidates for hearing aids.

Figure 4.8 is a typical pure-tone audiogram of a male aged 70–80 with a sensorineural impairment due to presbyacusis. Here bone and air conduction thresholds are closely related, which, as already stated, is a characteristic of sensorineural loss.

The audiogram shows a sharp fall after 1,000 Hz in the higher frequencies. The practical effect is that while lower-pitched vowel sounds will still be audible, difficulty will be experienced

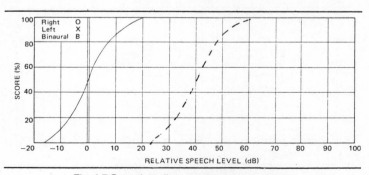

Fig. 4.7 Speech audiogram showing otosclerosis

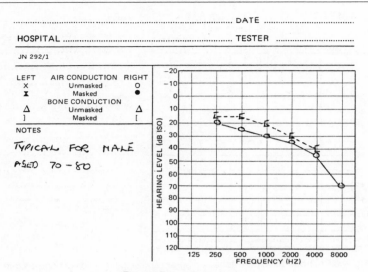

Fig. 4.8 Pure-tone audiogram

in hearing higher-pitched consonant sounds. Recruitment will adversely affect rehabilitation with a hearing aid.

Figure 4.9 is the speech audiogram of a person with a sensorineural loss. (Again, the speech discrimination curve for a person with normal hearing is shown on the left.) Not until the intensity level is raised to about 65 dB will 50 per cent of the words comprising the test be heard correctly. At between 75 dB and 90 dB the score improves to approximately 62 per cent. After this point discrimination deteriorates as amplification increases;

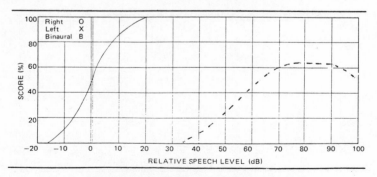

Fig. 4.9 Speech audiogram showing sensorineural loss

thus if the intensity level is raised to 95 dB the score declines to about 55 per cent. Parabolic curves are never found in pure conductive losses; they do, however, illustrate the effect of recruitment and the importance of considering this factor when prescribing hearing aids.

References

1   See Bennett, M. J. and Wade, K. H. 'Computerised Hearing Test for Neonates', *Hearing Aid Journal*, September 1981, pp.10, 52, 53.
2   DHSS Advisory Committee on Services for Hearing Impaired People. *Final Report of the Sub-Committee appointed to consider Services for Hearing Impaired Children*, ISBN 902 650 27 0, June 1981.
3   DHSS. *Prevention in the Child Health Services*, March 1980.
4   Taylor, I. Professor. *Paper given to a Conference on the Problems of Deaf People*, 9 February 1977.
5   Anderson. 'Hearing Screening for children', Katz (Ed), *Handbook of Clinical Audiology*, 2nd Ed., Ch. 5, p.52. Williams and Wilkins, 1978.
6   International Labour Office. 'Protection of Workers against Noise and Vibration in the Working Environment', *ILO Code of Practice*, 1980.

Chapter 5

Some communication, psychological and social problems of deaf, deafened and hard of hearing persons

An understanding of the possible consequences of hearing loss is essential for all who may be concerned with the rehabilitation of hearing impaired persons. This chapter deals with three important areas: namely, the effects of hearing loss on verbal communication, and some psychological and social consequences of hearing impairment.

Verbal communication

All persons with a significant hearing loss experience difficulties with verbal communication. There is, however, a profound distinction between the communication problems of a prelingually deaf person and one who has been deafened after the acquisition of speech and language.

Speech and language are naturally acquired through hearing. At first a normal child has only a general awareness of sound. Soon particular sounds are associated with specific persons or objects and stored in the speech centres of the brain. After a few months a baby uses this store of auditory sensations initially for his own pleasure in gurgling and cooing and later to imitate words that he often hears. By 2 years of age the vocalisation of 'dadadada' all have become shortened to 'dada', a meaningful oral symbol for a person. Later two or three words will be combined into phrases and sentences. By the time the child is 6, language pattern will have become established. This will include the correct articulation of sounds and a facility with language which will correspond closely to that constantly heard. In this way national languages and provincial pecularities and identities are perpetuated. Other elements such as pitch, quality, loudness, tone, rhythm and stress which, with articulation, combine to make up speech will also have been acquired.

In contrast, a born deaf or early deafened child deprived of the sound of the human voice is 'deaf, dumb and wordless'. To remedy this situation, special educational procedures must be used but several difficulties relating to communication have to be overcome. Although vision and amplification of residual hearing are harnessed to develop speech, vocabulary building is retarded. Other language problems are those involving word order, words with multiple meanings, abstract concepts and the use of plurals, pronouns and verb tenses.

Even after acquisition the intelligibility of speech may be affected by faulty articulation and modulation due to the inability of a deaf child to monitor its own voice. Markides[1] asked two panels of assessors, the first comprising teachers of the deaf, the second, university students without special knowledge of hearing impairment, to judge for intelligibility, the descriptions of five pictures by 58 deaf and 27 partially hearing children. 'Intelligibility' for this experiment was defined as the number of words understood as a percentage of the total words spoken. In an articulation test, the deaf children misarticulated 56 per cent of all vowels and 72 per cent of the consonants. The scores for intelligibility by the teachers and students were 31 per cent and 19 per cent respectively, suggesting that those unaccustomed to working with the profoundly deaf have greater difficulty than specialists in understanding their speech. Markides reported that intelligibility declined with the severity of the impairment and improved slightly for older children.

With older children and adults the need to acquire speech and language does not, of course, arise although the difficulties of verbal communication are still present. Three factors affecting these difficulties are the type and severity of the hearing loss, the effect on speech and the isolation which limited participation in social intercourse may impose. Apart from surgical rehabilitation, a pure conductive impairment may often be almost completely overcome by amplification using a suitable hearing aid. With a sensorineural impairment a hearing aid is of less benefit due to diminished speech discrimination and the effect of recruitment.

Background noise occuring, for example, during meals or at a station, causes difficulty in comprehending speech in group situations. Similar difficulties can be caused by the way different furnishings affect the acoustics, e.g. hard versus carpeted floors or soft-cushioned furnishings compared with those made from hard wood or metal.

With a profound loss, say of over 90 dB in the better ear, speech and articulation may deteriorate. Conscious of poor speech and of his inability to modulate his voice, a hearing impaired person may be reluctant to speak. In such cases, speech therapy involving speech improvement and conservation is required.

Finally, as Rawson says,[2] the inability to understand speech in the normal conditions of everyday life:

results in a considerable degree of isolation, particularly in our society with its increasingly ambient noise and the widespread use of recorded sound – e.g. radio and television for news and leisure activities and the use of telephones instead of letters.

This isolation is an important influence in the psychological adjustment of the hearing impaired person.

Psychological consequences

There is an immense literature relating to the psychological consequences of hearing impairment. In evaluating statements relating to the psychology of hearing loss, four facts must be remembered:

1 While generalisations regarding the effects of hearing loss can be made, every hearing impaired person must be regarded as an individual and not stereotyped.

2 The type of test administered and the knowledge of hearing impairment and ability of the investigator to communicate with the deaf should be considered when evaluating the results of intelligence and personality studies relating to hearing impaired persons, particularly the pre-lingually deaf.

3 The response to hearing loss of any individual will be influenced by many variables relating to the impairment, especially the age of onset and its severity, together with personal, educational and social factors.

4 There are profound differences in the responses of the pre-

lingually deaf, the traumatically deafened and the hard of hearing.

The pre-lingually deaf

At birth a deaf child has the same psychological needs as one who hears. Intelligence and personality, both influenced by the interplay from birth onwards of inherited and environmental factors, will be unaffected by the hearing impairment. The factor that will most profoundly retard subsequent development is the limited ability to make auditory contact with the environment and especially the extent to which verbal communication is restricted.

From the outset, two factors, the mother–child relationship and the attitudes of the parents to the child, will have important consequences.

If either mother or child is deaf, communication with the other is limited. Only a few weeks after birth, a baby can be quieted by the sound of its mother's voice even if she is in another room. When the child is deaf this intimate auditory contact between mother and child is lost. This effect can be minimised if, without over-indulging, the mother has time to devote to the child. The adjustment will be helped if, during the formative years, parents can learn to communicate with the child, not only through speech but also by tactile and visual means.

The child's intellectual and social development will also be influenced according to whether parents display an attitude of acceptance or rejection and the extent to which they are prepared to obtain an understanding of the consequences of hearing loss.

It is dangerous to attempt to summarise the results of research findings with regard to the intelligence, personalities and adjustment of pre-lingually deaf children and adults. Three statements would, however, probably receive the endorsement of the majority of workers in this field.

1 The educational development of pre-lingually deaf persons compared with the hearing is retarded. This does not mean that the deaf are of lower mental ability but that they are handicapped by the need to acquire language as a preliminary to learning. Achievement will probably be lowest in areas dependent on the understanding and use

of English and highest where non-verbal skills and abilities are required.

2   Many generalisations have been made regarding the effects of pre-lingual hearing loss on personality. With deaf children Levine[3] identified such characteristics as egocentricity, easy irritability, impulsiveness and suggestibility. Altshuler[4] added dependency and lack of empathy. These traits have also been applied to deaf adults with the addition of others such as introversion, despondency, hopelessness, persecution complex, cruelty and lack of sympathy. Evidence has been adduced that deaf persons are prone to paranoia and schizophrenia. While it seems likely that there is some substance in these findings, it is important to remember the precautions in evaluating such statements made earlier in this chapter. Psychiatrists who have little experience of the deaf may, for example, wrongly diagnose a deaf person as schizophrenic on the basis of poor language ability. Myklebust,[5] using the Minnesota Multiphase Personality Inventory, found a schizophrenic tendency in his sample of deaf persons but recommended caution in the interpretation of his results, suggesting that they did not necessarily mean that the deaf are schizophrenic but, that compared with the hearing, they feel more detached and isolated from other people. Similarly the paranoid stereotype probably applies less to the deaf than the deafened and hard of hearing who, feeling that they are missing things, may become suspicious and embarrassed.

3   Myklebust reported that while the deaf showed greater emotional disorder than the hard of hearing, they were largely unaware of deafness as a handicap. Since they have never consciously experienced themselves as hearing persons, the pre-lingually deaf generally adjust better to their impairment than the deafened and hard of hearing. The pre-lingually deaf have not the consciousness of losing a faculty once possessed or comparing their previous experience of hearing and their present situation as hearing impaired persons.

The deafened

As McCall[6] states: 'Sudden bilateral profound deafness in adult life presents a totally different situation from pre-lingual deafness, deafness in childhood or from that of people who can benefit from amplified sound.' The psychological shock of sudden profound loss will result in feelings of fear and loneliness similar to that of bereavement and a feeling of 'deadness'. This 'deadness' is explained by Ramsdell,[7] who identified three psychological functions of hearing: the 'primitive', the 'warning' and the 'symbolic'. The primitive function refers to undifferentiated background noise to which we give no attention unless our attention is consciously aroused. Thus, it is only when I *listen* that I am aware of the traffic outside my window. The warning level refers to sounds that are signals to action such as a fire alarm. The most complex level of hearing is the use of sounds as symbols for the purpose of communication as when we transmit and receive messages by speech. Ramsdell believes that the depression consequent on the loss of hearing is due to the loss of hearing at the primitive rather than the symbolic level since the person is cut off from auditory contact with his environment. These feelings of depression are often enhanced by social factors. Some such factors relating to the deafened (which depending on the severity of the impairment also affect the hard of hearing) have been identified by McCall:[6]

1 The diminished opportunities for conversation and the embarrassment of misunderstandings.
2 Missing the tone of voice which conveys so much.
3 The humiliation of being thought stupid.
4 The impossibilities of easy participation in discussions, groups, meetings, committees, lectures.
5 The depreciation of verbal wit and repartee.
6 The fatigue caused by constant alertness – to maintain communication the concentration needed is very demanding.
7 The depreciation of social information from which to select, evaluate and formulate opinions and assess the social mood.
8 The inability to do 2 things at the same time (eat and lip read, for example).
9 The reasons for decisions not being clearly understood; being excluded from decision-making. 'I'll tell you afterwards' is no use. 'Afterwards' is too late to participate.
10 The lack of stimulation of discussion and debate, the sharpening of mind on mind.
11 The uncertainty caused when people act unexpectedly without explanations.

12   The enormous difficulties of previously simple encounters, such as dealing with the gas men who won't write things down and cannot be lip-read.

13   The risk of paranoid feelings and the reality of being left out.

The hard of hearing

The pre-lingually profoundly deaf person has little or no experience of hearing while the traumatically deafened person has suffered a sudden deprivation of sound. In contrast, a person with an irreversible progressive loss, while having a longer period in which to adjust, has also to cope with misunderstanding and the anxiety of contemplating the possible consequences of progressively deteriorating hearing on employment and social relationships and on the ability to cope with any situation requiring auditory cues or response.

Because the impairment is insidious in its onset and may progress through the stages of slight, moderate and severe, both hard of hearing children and adults may have to cope with misunderstanding from their families, teachers, employers and other associates. The child will be accused of slowness and inattentiveness, the adult of being unsociable and withdrawn. While the intelligence of the child will be unaffected, educational progress may be adversely affected. Psychological reactions to progressive hearing impairment include anxiety, anger, apathy, dependency, exaggeration of symptoms, frustration, self-centredness and submissiveness. The hearing impaired person may resort to such defence mechanisms as denial of the impairment, withdrawal from society, over-compensation and self-rejection. These reactions will be strongly influenced by the basic personality of the individual.

Thomas[8] surveyed the effects of severe hearing loss on personality using the Eysenck Personality Questionnaire with a sample of adults of employment age (up to 64 for men and 59 for women) living in the Greater London area with a sensorineural loss of 60 dB or greater averaged across the speech frequencies. He concluded that 'while hearing loss is known to be highly stressful and associated with psychological disturbance at the psychoneurotic level' there was no evidence of personality change and that 'hearing loss is unlikely to result in a greater likelihood of paranoid illness'. Not all researchers would wholly endorse these views. Myklebust,[5] after comparing the reaction of deaf and hard of hearing persons, stated that 'deafness, particularly when profound and from early life imposes a characteristic restriction on personality but does not cause mental illness'. From his study of 127 hard of hearing persons (44 men and 83 women) with average age and hearing loss of 45 years and 67 dB respectively, Myklebust reported the following findings:

1   Better adjustment was associated with the use of a hearing aid.
2   There was no evidence of suspiciousness by his subjects.
3   Married women adjusted better than those who were single or divorced.
4   Older females adjusted better.
5   Better adjustment was associated with higher educational attainment.
6   In general females showed less emotional maladjustment than males.

While such researches help in understanding deaf, deafened and hard of hearing persons, the danger of making generalisations on the basis of isolated studies of the psychological effects of hearing impairment must be reiterated.

Social consequences

Effective rehabilitation of a person with hearing loss requires an understanding not only of the sensory impairment and its psychological consequences but also of the sociological implications for its owner. A person with a hearing loss is socially handicapped in two ways: firstly, by the restricted opportunities imposed by loss of hearing for contact with the environment; secondly, by the attitudes of hearing persons to the impairment and the effects of such attitudes on the self-image of an individual. When considering the social consequences of hearing loss, it is important to distinguish between those for the deaf and those for the deafened and hard of hearing. In both cases the concepts of deviance, stigma and marginality will apply.

Deviance refers to behaviour which infringes rules or the expectations of others and which attracts disapproval or punishment. Being identified as deviant places a person in a new status and thus has profound consequences for the individual who will become labelled or stereotyped.

Stigma is defined by Goffman[9] as 'an attribute that is deeply discrediting' or 'an undesired differentness' from what has been expected by 'normals'.

Marginality is a term used mainly in the context of race and nationality to describe a person who belongs to two cultural worlds and will experience tension because he is fully integrated into neither.

How these concepts may be applied to deaf and deafened or hard of hearing persons is briefly considered below.

Deaf persons

The pre-lingually profoundly deaf person may be regarded as deviant for at least two reasons. Firstly an important factor in deviance, particularly when the deviance arises from an impairment, is visibility. Hearing impairment, unlike blindness, is invisible until a deaf person has to communicate. In this situation the use of signs will identify him as different while as Thouless says[10] 'The characteristic loud and monotonous speech of a deaf child or adult may be interpreted either as a mark of imbecility or when it occurs less strikingly as a personality defect which leads the individual concerned to draw attention to himself.'

Secondly pre-lingual deafness retards not only educational development but maturation. Levine[11] specifies five qualifications as essential to the attainment of social adequacy and maturity, namely:

1 Information about social habits, customs and usage.
2 Ample experience in putting such information to use.
3 Sufficient opportunities to enjoy a wide range of social and inter-personal relationships.
4 Attitudes that will impel a person to seek such experience.
5 A healthy psychic structure that will provide wholesome, well-balanced motivation.

These qualifications apply equally to both hearing and deaf persons but as Levine goes on to say[11]

The important difference stems from the fact that the deaf are more vulnerable to adverse influences by reason of the situations that auditory disability creates. Language is more difficult to come by for the deaf; experiences and opportunities for social contact are more limited; attitudes needed for gaining a foothold in hearing society require intense cultivation; and the developing psychic structure is subject to greater hazards when one is deaf. It follows, therefore, that social maturity is also more difficult to attain for a deaf person than a hearing one.

Backwardness and lack of maturity by deaf persons in dealing with social and personal problems may be attributed by the uninformed to deviant behaviour rather than the true cause which is a restricted life experience.

Stigma with its associated labelling derives from deviance. The deaf person who signs is still likely to be labelled deaf and dumb even though this term is obsolete. The hearing are also likely to have lower expectations of the deaf. Prejudice towards the deaf, as with all disabled, is exhibited by consistently negative prejudgements and behaviour which emphasise devaluation and rejection of an impaired person. The expression 'dummy', stated by Partridge[12] to be a colloquialism applied to the deaf in the sixteenth century and which by the end of the seventeenth century had acquired the meaning of 'notably deficient in ability and brightness', is indicative of the popular belief that the deaf were of subnormal intelligence. How this belief persists is exemplified by Gorman,[13] a man born with no useful hearing, who obtained the degree of Doctor of Philosophy at Cambridge. Gorman shows how a hearing individual may meet a deaf person who can speech-read and carry on an adequate conversation.

Because of his peculiar voice, his slightly imperfect English and more than ordinary use of hand gestures, the deaf person may be mistaken for a foreigner and the conversation is governed only by the attitude the hearing person holds for that type of foreigner. If later he discovers or is told that the so-called foreigner is deaf, there is a sudden and marked change in the conversation, the topics become more trivial, much simpler words are used and the hearing person may either close the conversation very soon or turn his attention to other hearing persons in the group. He thus ignores the deaf person.

Marginality with the pre-lingual deaf may arise from different concepts of the rehabilitation process. The aim of educators of the deaf who stress oral methods is the integration of their pupils into the hearing community. Complete integration is, however, rarely achieved due to the isolating nature of the impairment itself and the failure of many pupils to acquire a level of speech and literacy necessary for social competency. Integration, in any event, is a two-way process and the general attitude of the hearing towards the profoundly deaf is coloured by amusement, charity, impatience, pity and sympathy so that though the deaf are generally tolerated they are rarely 'fully accepted'.

Three possible social roles are therefore open to the deaf person. At one extreme he may try to function entirely within the hearing community and reject the deaf community. At the other extreme he may function within the deaf community and reject the hearing community so far as he is allowed to do by economic and geographical conditions. A third possibility is for a deaf person to function according to his needs and preferences in both the deaf and hearing communities. It is in this last situation that he is likely to experience marginality.

Deafened and hard of hearing persons

These two categories of hearing impairment may be considered together since, as stated in the following quotation,[14] they differ from the pre-lingual deaf in having to make the transition from normality to abnormality.

Between the psychological attitudes of the deaf and the deafened (or hard of hearing) there is an almost unbridgeable gulf. It must be emphasised that at the beginning of their lives the deaf are abnormals shut off from that stream of verbally conveyed ideas which moulds the individual mind to general sameness with the mental pattern of society and throughout their lives the deaf are abnormals struggling towards full normalcy. The deafened on the other hand are normals threatened with all the horror of abnormalcy. To the change in their state and particularly the change in the behaviour of other people towards them, they are particularly sensitive . . . they will not class themselves with the 'true deaf' nor will they approach deaf organisations for help. They are thus a class apart.

When a person becomes deafened or hard of hearing he or she is likely to become acutely aware of the extent of deviance from the norm and the stigmatising consequence of the impairment. An individual may shrink from wearing a hearing aid because this 'advertises the disability'. There may, as stated above, be a refusal to seek help since this would mean being identified with a stigmatised group. The feeling of stigma is likely to be re-inforced by negative attitudes on the part of people with normal hearing such as discrimination in employment or promotion situations or a change in social status or traditional roles. As one hard of hearing man remarked to the writer, 'If we have burglars my wife will have to get up because I shan't hear them.'

Because of such feelings of stigma it is not surprising that the deafened and the hard of hearing may attempt to pass as normal. While a deafened person cannot for long hide the impairment, a person with a progressive hearing loss may deny the disability: 'I'm not deaf', refuse to wear a hearing aid and attempt to pass as normal by resorting to subterfuges such as simulated pre-occupation or absentmindedness.

Marginality is more likely to affect people who become deafened or profoundly hard of hearing than the pre-lingually deaf since, as Sussman[15] observes, the latter are in a better position to adjust because they accept their hearing deficiency and have taken on new techniques which do not require the auditory process. They do not therefore face the problems of marginality characterising the deafened or profoundly hard of hearing person who may fluctuate between the world of the deaf and that of the hearing.

References

1   Markides, A. 'The Speech of Deaf and Partially Hearing Children with Special Reference to Factors affecting intelligibility', *British Journal of Disorders of Communication*, Vol. 5, 1970, pp.126–140.
2   Rawson, Annette. *Deafness: Report of a Departmental Enquiry and the Promotion of Research*, DHSS, published by HMSO, 1973, Ch. 3, p.21.
3   Levine, E. *Youth in a Soundless World. A Search for Personality*, New York University Press, 1956.
4   Altshuler, K. 'Psychiatric Considerations in the Adult Deaf', *American Annals of the Deaf*, Vol. 107, pp.560–561, 1962.
5   Myklebust, H. R. 'The Psychological Effects of Deafness', *American Annals of the Deaf*, Vol. 105, pp.372–385, 1960.
6   McCall, R. F. 'The Effects of Sudden Profound Hearing Loss in Adult Life', Paper given to the British Society of Audiology, 10 July 1981.
7   Ramsdell D. A. 'The Psychology of the Hard of Hearing and Deafened Adult', *Hearing and Deafness*, Davis H. and Silverman, S. (Eds.), 4th Edition, Holt, Rinehart and Winston, 1978.
8   Thomas, A. J. 'The Effect of Severe Hearing Loss on Personality', *Social and Occupational Medicine*, Vol. 9, 1981, pp.941–942.
9   Goffman, E. G. *Stigma*, Pelican Books, 1968, Ch. 1, p.13.
10 Thouless. 'Social Psychological Problems of the Handicapped Individual', *Teacher of the Deaf*, Vol. 55, Oct. 1957, pp.162–164.
11 Levine, E. S. 'Psychological Aspects and Problems of Early Profound Deafness, *American Annals of the Deaf*, Vol. 103, March 1958, p.338.

12 Partridge, E. *Dictionary of Slang*.
13 Gorman, P. P. 'Deaf People in a Hearing Society', Paper presented to the British Association for the Advancement of Science, Oxford, 1954.
14 Evans, J. D. 'Voluntary Organisations for the Welfare of the Deaf', *Voluntary Social Services – Their Place in the Modern State*, Bourdillon (Ed.), Methuen, 1945, pp.73–74.
15 Sussman. *Sociological Theory and Deafness. Problems and Prospects In Research on Behavioural Aspects of Deafness*, US Department of Health, Education and Welfare, 1965.

Chapter 6

Aural rehabilitation

Aural rehabilitation is a general term for those measures designed to remove or ameliorate the disabilities or handicaps consequent on hearing impairment. Strictly, rehabilitation refers to acquired hearing loss. Measures for the assistance of the pre-lingually deaf are properly described as 'habilitation' since it is not possible to restore something that has never existed. In practice the words 'rehabilitation' and 'habilitation' are used interchangeably.

The concept of a comprehensive rehabilitation service for the hearing impaired is difficult to define. As the DHSS Advisory Committee on Services for Hearing Impaired People[1] observed:

The needs of each individual will vary according to the degree of hearing loss, the time and type of onset and individual circumstances. In its entirety, the process of rehabilitation should involve the use of a number of skills which should ideally be provided (but at present are not) in consequence by the services of the otolaryngologist, scientific audiologist, physiological measurement technician (audiology), social worker and a worker suitably trained to give lipreading instruction, auditory training and speech correction. In some instances part of the process may be provided by people from other disciplines – such as a psychiatrist, psychologist, health visitor or disablement resettlement officer. Furthermore the special problems and needs of the hearing impaired may involve discussions with and help from family members, neighbours and employers or teachers; and that to help educate society about what is needed, the informed interest of the media must be encouraged.

The DHSS report from which the above extract is taken referred to 'the adult hearing impaired with an acquired loss'. In this context rehabilitation was defined as 'enabling anyone with an acquired deafness to lead as far as possible an independent life within the community' and 'the core of the rehabilitation process' to be the follow-up of patients attending the ENT Department of a hospital. This approach ignores the problems both in childhood and adulthood of the pre-lingually deaf. It was, in fact, in this area that aural habilitation began, firstly through the efforts of teachers of the deaf who were concerned with developing speech and language and secondly by 'missioners' or welfare officers associated with voluntary societies who endeavoured to cater for the material and spiritual needs of deaf persons in adult life. The rehabilitation of persons with an acquired loss received little attention until after World War II.

Disciplines concerned with hearing impairment

Rawson,[2] writing in 1973, identified 20 different disciplines involved in hearing *research*. From the standpoint of *rehabilitation*, however, the main occupations concerned with hearing impairment are stated below.

Audiological scientist is a term applied to a graduate scientist in audiology responsible to a consultant otolaryngologist or audiological physician for selecting and carrying out audiological and vestibular tests and reporting the results; the training of other staff in audiology, including the training of other staff in audiology, the rehabilitation of hearing impaired patients and the management within a prescribed area of audiological services.

Audiological physicians are medical practitioners concerned with the diagnosis, medical treatment and rehabilitation of patients with auditory and vestibular disorders. The speciality was officially recognised in 1975 when the Joint Committee on Higher Medical Training defined a formal training programme. The British Association of Audiological Physicians was formed in April 1977 to bring together consultants working predominantly in the field of audiological medicine.[3]

Audiological technicians. See *Physiological measurement technician (audiology).*

Developmental paediatricians as medical practitioners are involved in the diagnosis of hearing impairment and other communication disorders in children.

Educational audiologists are concerned with the preliminary audiometric assessment of school children, the placing, in consultation with a medical practitioner employed in the school medical service or community medicine, of the child in a suitable educational environment, help to parents and often some of the duties described below under 'Psychologists'.

General practitioners are often the first point of reference for persons with an actual or suspected hearing impairment. The attitude of the general practitioner to hearing impairment may have a significant influence on rehabilitation. If this is dismissive or uninformed for example, the patient may not seek help or wrongly conclude that nothing can be done. In all cases of doubt a patient should therefore be referred to a consultant otologist or audiological physician.

Health visitors frequently undertake the preliminary screening of babies for hearing and may be the first to recognise abnormal development in a baby.

Hearing Aid Dispensers are employed by commercial organisations to prescribe and sell hearing aids (see Chapter 10).

Hearing therapists work within the National Health Service to assess and, so far as possible, provide for the medical, technical, social, financial, environmental, vocational and educational needs of hearing impaired persons from a rehabilitative standpoint (see Chapter 10).

Lip or speech-reading teachers give lip or speech-reading instruction to adults with a hearing loss.

Consultant otologists are medical specialists responsible for the diagnosis of hearing impairment and, where applicable, for its surgical treatment.

Physiological measurement technicians, (audiology), PTM(A)S, formerly known as audiology technicians or audiometricians, may, under the direction of an audiological scientist, audiological physician or consultant otologist undertake a range of audiometric and vestibular tests and the selection and fitting of hearing aids (see Chapter 10).

Psychiatrists, particularly those who can communicate with pre-lingually deaf persons and others with an acquired hearing loss, are needed to help with the psychiatric problems which arise owing to the difficulties of normal communication (see Chapter 8).

Psychologists may be clinical or educational and are concerned with the initial diagnosis, assessment and training of children, their school placement, social and educational progress, vocational training and emotional problems. The educational psychologist is particularly concerned with remedial teaching.

Social workers may be concerned with the personal and family problems of hearing impaired persons.

Social workers with the deaf may be employed either by a local authority social services department or a voluntary society to provide specialist help in those cases of hearing impairment where a knowledge of the psychology of hearing loss and the ability to communicate by manual or total communication methods is essential (see Chapter 8).

Speech therapists are mainly concerned with the conservation of speech with the hard of hearing and deafened adults.

Teachers of the deaf are specially trained to teach deaf children and, in the case of peripatetic teachers, to give guidance to parents.

The organisation of services for the hearing impaired

The above range of specialisms indicates the need for multi-disciplinary approach to rehabilitation. A DHSS sub-committee appointed to consider the needs of hearing impaired children[4] suggested that a team of workers might comprise:

a consultant otologist or consultant in audiological medicine, a senior clinical medical officer, a clinical or educational psychologist, a health visitor or school nurse, a teacher of the deaf, an audiological scientist, a physiological measurement technician (audiology), a speech therapist and a social worker with special training.

Much the same team, would, ideally, be involved with the rehabilitation of hearing impaired adults. Since rehabilitation is concerned with the whole person, it is likely to be less than satisfactory where an individual specialist tries to provide a service in isolation from other workers. Decision-making with regard to the rehabilitation needs of an individual is likely to be more comprehensive and relevant when contributions from members of a case conference or reports from others concerned with the client have the information regarding the areas identified below.

1 *Personal information.* Furnished by the client via a question-
    naire or an interview with a social worker or hearing

therapist, this relates to age, age of onset of hearing impairment, marital state, general and vocational education and training, present and previous employment, interests and hobbies, perceived reactions to hearing loss on the part of the client, his or her family and the community.

2 *General health information.* Furnished by the client's general practitioner or obtained by medical examination, this information is important because hearing and rehabilitation measures may be affected by the client's general health and such factors as poor eyesight or arthritic conditions which may respectively affect speech-reading ability or cause difficulty in operating the controls of a hearing aid.

3 *Audiological information.* Furnished by the otologist, audiological physician or audiological scientist, this data is derived from audiometric, vestibular and other tests regarding the nature, cause, severity and likely progress of the client's hearing loss. It will provide the focus for all other information and is the starting point for all rehabilitative measures.

4 *Psychological/psychiatric information.* Furnished, where appropriate, by a psychologist or psychiatrist, it can give useful insights into factors that influence the effectiveness of rehabilitation measures such as the client's intelligence, personality, attitudes and aptitudes. Manifestations of emotionally disturbed behaviour include nervousness, irritation over minor matters, defensiveness, suspicion, lack of confidence, over-confidence, over-compensation and unfriendliness. Projective tests may be useful with some hard of hearing persons to provide an objective evaluation that can be shared with the client to the extent that this is desirable. In many cases personality rehabilitation and the fostering of a constructive attitude to the disability is essential before assistance in other areas can be successfully provided.

5 *Social information.* Furnished by a social worker or hearing therapist, this can provide particulars of the client's socio-economic status, family acceptance and attitudes to the client's hearing loss and community services and facilities that can be made available.

6 *Vocational information.* Furnished by a specialist in vocational counselling or disablement resettlement officer, it relates to the extent to which the client's occupational experience, interests and qualifications can be utilised; to opportunities

for retraining and available aids that can assist the client to cope with the handicaps consequent on his disability.

Other useful data can be furnished by such workers as the *speech therapist* (speech intelligibility and voice control) and the *teacher of speech-reading* (aptitude for speech-reading and auditory training) where appropriate specially-devised tests may be utilised such as the scales for hearing handicap, social handicap and hearing measurement referred to in Chapter 4.

Case conferences along the above lines are exceptional in the field of aural rehabilitation. The DHSS sub-committee appointed 'To Consider the Role of the Social Services in the Care of the Deaf of All Ages' (1977) stated that in only very few areas had an attempt been made to co-ordinate services in respect of the deaf child and his parents and emphasised that relatively little communication takes place between the medical and social services:

It is of fundamental importance that the social implications of deafness should be recognised by those responsible for diagnosis, and the fact that this is often not the case may be due, to some extent, to the limited emphasis on audiology in the basic medical training of doctors.[5]

An earlier sub-committee, in its report on 'The Rehabilitation of the Adult Hearing Impaired' (1975),[1] identified the main problem in this area as being the filling of the follow-up gap which occurs after a hearing aid is fitted and doubted whether, in view of the shortage of existing categories of all workers with the hearing impaired, a team approach would achieve the necessary rehabilitation. The appointment of a new category of worker – the hearing therapist – referred to earlier was therefore recommended.

Yet co-operation between workers in the field of hearing impairment is an aim to work for, and the following official policy statement of the British Society of Audiology[6] points the way:

Aural rehabilitation of hearing-impaired adults needs to be tackled in a systematic way as an integral service development: co-ordinated by Health Authorities and based both within the Community and at the local hearing aid clinic. The skeleton of such a future service is diagrammatically summarised in the following chart. [Fig. 6.1]

The same policy statement also draws attention to the need for heath authorities and other agencies to provide a range of

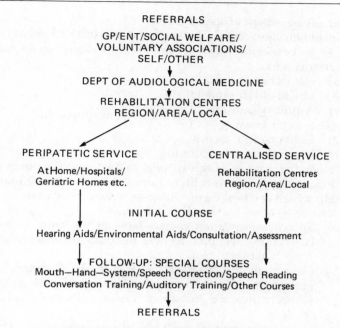

REFERRALS

GP/ENT/SOCIAL WELFARE/
VOLUNTARY ASSOCIATIONS/
SELF/OTHER

DEPT OF AUDIOLOGICAL MEDICINE

REHABILITATION CENTRES
REGION/AREA/LOCAL

PERIPATETIC SERVICE

AtHome/Hospitals/
Geriatric Homes etc.

CENTRALISED SERVICE

Rehabilitation Centres
Region/Area/Local

INITIAL COURSE

Hearing Aids/Environmental Aids/Consultation/Assessment

FOLLOW-UP: SPECIAL COURSES
Mouth—Hand—System/Speech Correction/Speech Reading
Conversation Training/Auditory Training/Other Courses

REFERRALS

ENT/Residential Rehabilitation Centre/Social Welfare
Multiple Handicap/Environmental Aids/Hearing Aids
GP/Church/Voluntary Associations/Disablement Resettlement Officers/
Further Education/Other

Fig. 6.1 Organisation chart 1 of aural rehabilitation services
(British Society of Audiology)

courses designed to assist hearing impaired persons and, where appropriate, their families.

Such courses fall into the following four categories:

1 *Information courses.* Of one or two sessions each of one to two hours for all new patients issued with a hearing aid, they are designed to include fundamental information on:

(a) Deafness (pathology, type, severity, treatment etc.).

(b) Hearing aid use (advantages, limitations, basic maintenance, manipulation etc.).

(c) Environmental aids (availability, demonstration, use etc.).

(d) Communication tactics (audio-visual approach, positioning, monitoring speech loudness, tackling different communication situations etc.).

(e) Assessment of special needs.
2 *Communication courses.* Extending over 8 to 12 weeks at from one to two hours each week, they are designed to assist patients with:
(a) Use of hearing aid.
(b) Use of environmental aids.
(c) Auditory training ⎱ Audio-visual approach.
(d) Speech-reading ⎰
(e) Conversation tactics.
(f) Psycho-social functioning.
3 *Residential courses.* Lasting one to two months, they are designed for patients who require substantial rehabilitative help which can best be provided on a residential basis.
4 *Other specialised courses.* These include:
(a) *Speech conservation courses* (speech teaching – speech correction) designed to help the patient conserve good speech habits.
(b) *Courses in the Mouth–Hand System.* In Denmark this system has been found to offer substantial help to severely hearing impaired adults with their speech-reading.
(c) *Courses in manual methods of communication.* These courses relate primarily to pre-lingually severely deaf adults but it may be that a small number of deafened adults will find such courses of some use.

References

1 DHSS, *Report of a Sub-Committee appointed to consider the Rehabilitation of the Adult Hearing Impaired*, September 1975.
2 Rawson, A. *Deafness: Report of a Departmental Enquiry into the Promotion of Research, Reports on Health and Social Subjects, No. 4.,* DHSS, HMSO, 1973.
3 Stephens, S. D. G., 'Existence and Role of Audiological Physicians', *Hospital Update*, Nov. 1978, pp.701–707.
4 DHSS. *Final Report of the Sub-Committee appointed to Consider Services for Hearing Impaired Children,* June 1981.
5 DHSS *Report of a Sub-Committee appointed to consider the Role of Social Services in the Care of the Deaf of all Ages,* June 1977.
6 Markides, A. Brooks, D. N. Hart, F. G. and Stephens, S. D. G. 'Rehabilitation of Hearing Impaired Adults (Policy of the British Society of Audiology)', *British Journal of Audiology*, 1979, Vol. 13, pp.7–14.

Chapter 7

Hearing impaired children and young persons

The rehabilitation problems of a hearing impaired child are complex and in a general book only a brief consideration of such important issues as educational assessment, educational provision, further education and employment is possible.

Educational assessment

Section 1 of the Education Act 1981 implements the recommendation of the Warnock Committee that the 1944 Act system of special educational treatment for pupils suffering from a disability of mind or body who were classified in specified categories of handicap should be replaced by a concept of special education provision based on the *special educational needs* of individual children. A child has special educational needs if he has a learning difficulty which requires special educational provision to be made to meet those needs. 'Learning difficulty' means not only physical and mental difficulties, but 'any kind of learning difficulty experienced by a child provided that it is significantly greater than that of the majority of children of the same age'.

Section 10 of the Act requires health authorities to inform parents and the appropriate local education authority (LEA) of their opinion that a child under 5 has or is likely to have special educational needs. Discussions with the parents must precede notification to the LEA. Health authorities are also required to inform the parents of babies and young children if they think a voluntary organisation is likely to provide advice or assistance relating to the special educational needs of the child. The initiative for assessment may come from the LEA or the parent.

Section 4 of the Act makes LEAs responsible for the identification of special educational needs for all children in their areas who are at a maintained school or for whom the LEAs are providing education at a non-maintained or independent school or who have been brought to their attention as possibly having special educational needs. This duly extends to all children aged between 2 and 16 or 19 in respect of registered pupils at school. Under Section 6 of the Act, LEAs are empowered to assess the educational needs of children aged under 2 with the consent of the parents and are required to make an assessment where this is required by the parents.

Apart from children under 2 years the rules for the conduct of assessments of individual children by LEAs for the purpose of determining the educational provision to be made are prescribed in Section 5 of the Act. Particular importance is attached to the close involvement of parents throughout the process of assessment and LEAs should ensure that parents are acquainted with their rights under the Act. Briefly these parental rights are:

1 To be given notification of the intention of the LEA to make an assessment and information relating to the assessment procedure.
2 To make representations to the LEA within a period of not less than 29 days.
3 To be notified of the LEA's decision whether to proceed with the assessment, and, following assessment, whether to make a statement under Section 7 of the Act.
4 To be provided with the name of an officer of the LEA from whom further information may be obtained.
5 To be acquainted with their right of appeal to the Secretary of State if the LEA decide after assessment not to determine the special educational provision to be made for the child.

After an assessment the LEA may decide to make a statement relating to the special educational needs of the individual child. Parents must receive a draft of the proposed statement and be simultaneously informed of their rights to make representations within a 15-day period and to seek an interview with an officer of the LEA and subsequently, if desired, with some other person who has given advice with regard to the assessment or who is qualified to give such advice. If parents disagree with the statement issued by the LEA they may appeal successively to a local appeal committee and the Secretary of State.

LEAs are under a duty to arrange special educational provision in accordance with the statement as finally agreed.

Educational provision

Educational provision for hearing impaired persons covers the whole spectrum of pre-school, primary, secondary, further and higher education.

Pre-school education

Education begins at home. Soon after diagnosis and assessment the parents of a hearing impaired child should be visited by a peripatetic teacher of the deaf employed either by the health authority or the LEA. The main counselling roles of the peripatetic teacher are to help the parents accept their child's impairment, provide guidance in the management of hearing aids and attempt to involve the whole family in developing the child's speech and language. Most experts advise against too early placement in a play group or nursery class because initially the child needs the one-to-one attention and stimulation that will normally be best provided at home. Nursery classes may be available at some special schools but in most cases such classes for hearing impaired children are provided in ordinary schools.

Primary and secondary education

A key issue in the education of hearing impaired children, particularly those with a pre-lingual loss, is integration. Lynas[1] suggests that in deaf education 'the integration issue may perhaps have replaced the oral/manual debate as the central topic of controversy'. In actuality the aim of oral educators, whatever their successes, has always been to ensure that a deaf child should have the opportunity of developing the ability to communicate with hearing persons through speech and speech-reading and entering a wider world than the narrow, segregated one of deaf people only able to communicate by manual signs. Advances in hearing aids, the exploitation of residual hearing and the development of auditory training have led to increased emphasis on integration both as an educational and rehabilitative concept.

This emphasis is reflected in Section 2 of the 1981 Education Act which establishes the principle that all children for whom an LEA decides to make special educational provision are, so far as is reasonably practicable, to be educated in ordinary schools and associate in school activities with other children. This principle is subject to account having been taken of the views of the parents; the ability of the school to meet the child's special educational needs; the provision of efficient education for other children in the school and the efficient use of resources by the LEA. The Act also envisaged that from early 1982 maintained special schools would be discontinued. Educational provision at the pre-school, primary and secondary level may be broadly considered under the headings of provision in ordinary schools and special school provision.

Provision in ordinary schools

Many hearing impaired children can, with the assistance of a peripatetic or resident teacher of the deaf, cope as an individual member of a hearing class or as a member of a partially hearing unit (PHU) in an ordinary school. A PHU has been defined as: 'a group of partially hearing children which is being educated in any one school which has also children of normal hearing, and is under the care of one or more teachers of the deaf appointed for this purpose. A unit may consist of one class, several classes or a number of individual pupils distributed amongst the ordinary classes, who return to the special teacher for tutorial periods'. PHUs were first established in 1947 in four London primary schools for children considered capable of benefiting from the stimulus of listening to normal conversation, participating in main school lessons and activities and subsequently transferring according to the standard reached either to a normal class in an ordinary school or a special school for the partially hearing. A list obtainable from the RNID showed that in 1982 there were, in England, some 400 PHUs.

Lynas[2] has identified the following alleged educational advantages of placing a hearing impaired child in an ordinary school: a more stimulating learning environment; a wider curriculum than that normally offered in a special school; raised levels of expectations from associating with a greater variety of people with general higher standards of academic achievement. The social advantages of an ordinary school placement include:

better prospects of learning to adjust to life in the hearing community; residence at home rather than in a boarding school; an environment of natural, colloquial language in which confidence can be gained in the use of spoken language, fostering normal language development; normally hearing children possibly acquiring an understanding of hearing impairment.

The success of an individual placement in an ordinary school will depend partly on factors specific to the child such as the severity of loss and his propensity for developing oral skills and social competency and those relating to the environment, facilities, staffing and philosophy of the school. The latter group of factors include the use and provision of hearing aids, small groups, the quality of teachers – especially teachers of the deaf, the attitude of hearing pupils and good home/school liaison. The following guidelines are useful in relation to the admission of pupils to PHUs.[3]

1 In admitting children after the infant stage, care should be taken to select only those who function as partially hearing children.
2 They should be seen to have a prospect of learning to speak, with or without amplified sound, in a natural way more by listening than by lip-reading.
3 They should be capable of acquiring language along natural patterns rather than by the imposed patterns that are needed by the profoundly deaf.
4 In order to select children who collectively do not present too heavy a load of additional handicaps, the teacher of the unit should be consulted and should take part in all conferences.

Special schools

In England the numbers of maintained, non-maintained and independent special schools for the deaf and/or partially hearing listed by the DES in 1982 were 33, 13 and 6 respectively. The numbers of maintained special schools will however reduce due to falling rolls and the implementation of the 1981 Education Act. Sixteen maintained and all the non-maintained and residential schools catered for boarders; of the non-maintained establishments, six were wholly residential. A number of special schools provide all age education for pupils ranging from 2 to 19 years. The majority of special schools for hearing impaired children of secondary school age are of a general type and pupils are not selected according to ability or special aptitude. Two non-maintained schools which admit pupils who are specially selected on the basis of an entrance examination require special mention. The Mary Hare Grammar School for the Deaf, Newbury, Berkshire admits deaf and partially hearing boys and girls who show an aptitude for academic studies. The Burwood Park School, Walton-on-Thames is a secondary technical school for deaf boys. Both schools are residential and admit children from any part of the country who pass the entrance examination.

Although security and the development of speech and language are the most important factors in deciding whether a child attends a special school, other considerations include intelligence, speech-reading ability, auditory discrimination, personality and the quality of home support. The place of residence is also important. An LEA may decide that a child's educational needs may best be met by attending a school located in another authority. Many special schools for hearing impaired children now cater for pupils with other or additional physical, sensory or mental disabilities and placement in a residential school may be necessary either to obtain such special provision or the educational opportunities provided by the Mary Hare and Burwood Park schools.

Special schools claim such advantages as a concentration of specialised staff with an inclination towards working with hearing impaired children. They often work as a team with doctors, psychologists and others. It is true that 'through these skills and insights teachers and others in special schools are able to provide a combination of stimulating learning opportunities, specialised techniques, medical care and therapy and human relationships which have enabled many a handicapped child to develop his independence and resources to the fullest extent'.[4] A special school may provide a less stressful environment in which any consciousness of abnormalcy is minimised and the integration claimed from attendance at an ordinary school is often more apparent than real. A survey[5] of PHUs reported that while 'the facility in speech and conversational language achieved by partially hearing pupils . . . was 'commendable', comparable standards were seldom reached by pupils who were severely deaf'. Another statement in the same survey is important:

A significant number of parents were unaware of the quality of provision that is made in special schools. Some otologists and members of assessment teams in clinics were also resistant to education in special schools. There seemed to be confusion between assessing a child's ability to speak and assessing his capacity for learning in an ordinary speaking environment. For all these reasons, some children were kept in the units where the programme could never be related to their particular needs and the problems facing the teacher were thereby increased.

Placement should be regularly reviewed in the light of educational progress with the transfer, where appropriate, from one type of school to another. The ultimate consideration must be the well-being of the individual child.

Further and higher education

Success in further and higher education is largely dependent on the standards achieved at the primary and secondary stages. The majority of schools with hearing impaired secondary pupils provide courses leading to external examinations. Such courses may be provided either within the school or in collaboration with neighbouring hearing schools. Similarly, further education provision may be entirely within the school or in association with a local technical or art college. An example of the former is the Trade Training Department of the Royal Residential School for the Deaf, Manchester, where courses in catering and cabinet-making are offered for young people aged 16-18. Typical of the latter is the arrangement by which selected pupils from special schools for the hearing impaired in Birmingham attend part-time classes at the Matthew Boulton and Bournville Colleges of Further Education.

Some further education (FE) colleges have established special departments or sub-departments for hearing impaired students including adults. The largest of these is the Department of Further Education for the Deaf established by the Inner London Education Authority at the City Literary Institute, which, since 1975, has been a Regional Centre for Further Education of the Deaf. The aim of the Centre is 'to match the individual to a suitable course of FE whether it be at the Centre itself or in a modular course in conjunction with another college or as an individual placement at a college of further education, specialist college, polytechnic or college of higher education'. The centre offers a wide range of part-time, non-vocational courses and, in association with other colleges, full-time commercial and technical courses for hearing impaired young people. A full list, *Further Education Facilities for Hearing Impaired People* is obtainable from the RNID. A *Directory of Courses* is also available from The National Study Group on Further and Higher Education for the Hearing Impaired which has also published a *List of Concessions/Considerations for the Pre-Lingually Deaf in Public Examinations*. A useful booklet on FE is obtainable from the National Deaf Children's Society. The British Deaf Association offers a programme of non-vocational further education courses including practical activities such as skiing and pony-trekking and discussion groups dealing with leadership, current affairs, religion, ethics and similar subjects. Non-vocational FE courses which enable a hearing impaired person to become proficient at a craft or skill or to join in group activities can compensate to some extent for the social handicap consequent on the disability and has an important part to play in habilitation.

It is, however, the area of vocational preparation that is more important. Many hearing impaired school leavers are insufficiently prepared educationally, socially or emotionally for the world of employment according to their abilities and aptitudes. They need further education not only to obtain the qualifications to enter a particular type of employment but also to acquire the social and life skills necessary for independence in adult life.

Higher education poses considerable problems for the hearing impaired particularly the difficulty in following lectures and participating in tutorial discussion. A small number of students from Mary Hare Grammar School and Burwood Park School take degree or professional courses at universities or polytechnics. The Open University is doing some experimental work in the provision of higher education for the hearing impaired including special assistance with attendance at the residential summer school which is a compulsory element of some courses. Facilities for deaf students are also available at the College of St Hilda and St Bede of the University of Durham where a Tutor for Hearing Impaired Students has been appointed and a range of tutorial, note-taking, counselling and interpreting services instituted.

Careers guidance and employment

Careers guidance for hearing impaired pupils should be given during the last two years at school. Ideally careers guidance relates to three types of session.

1 Self-analysis sessions in which pupils are encouraged to come to terms with the handicap of hearing impairment and realistically appraise career possibilities in the light of interests, abilities and aptitudes.

2 Information sessions in which pupils are given particulars such as careers available especially in the locality of the school, opportunities of acquiring relevant qualifications, applying for jobs and behaviour at interviews. Guidance on such matters may be supplemented by industrial visits, work placements or link-courses at colleges of further education.

3 Sessions explaining the roles of careers teachers, careers officers and social workers for the deaf in finding placements or training and dealing with any subsequent difficulties.

The local authority careers service is responsible for providing vocational guidance and assistance in obtaining employment or training for all young people who seek help whether disabled or otherwise, and should, through school visits and reports, know all hearing impaired school leavers in its area. Information regarding school leavers from residential schools will be furnished to the home careers service of a pupil by a careers officer of the authority in which the school is located. With all hearing impaired pupils, particularly those who are profoundly deaf, the most satisfactory arrangement is for the careers teacher, careers officer and social worker for the deaf to combine as a team. A somewhat dated observation is still relevant.[6]

The interests of the child demand the mobilising of all available resources and no one, however experienced in work of this kind (youth employment) can afford to dispense with the specialised assistance of others.

Many deaf school leavers achieve too low an educational standard to obtain well-paid work or benefit greatly from further education opportunities. The decline in craftsmanship and the replacement of unskilled manual work by automation are also factors which are disadvantageous to the employment of deaf persons although it is possible that new occupations such as computer programming may offer employment to a minority of those of above-average educational attainment. Some other difficulties in securing employment, identified by the BDA, arise from the attitudes of employers, especially those relating to anticipated problems in communication and accident proneness due to inability to hear warning signals. The reason why many hearing impaired young workers are often underemployed and in dead-end jobs is largely because most employers regard simple, routine, low-skilled jobs as most 'suitable' for deaf and partially hearing persons. Such negative attitudes can be overcome only if, before leaving school, pupils have acquired a range of skill and competence necessary to enable them to compare favourably with their hearing contemporaries and make full use of their aptitudes.

References

1　Lynas, Wendy A. 'Integration and the Education of Hearing Impaired Children', *Journal British Association of Teachers of the Deaf*.
2　Lynas, Wendy. 'The Hearing-Impaired Child in the Ordinary School', *Teacher of the Deaf*, 1980, Vol. 4, pp.49–57.
3　Department of Education and Science. *Units for Partially Hearing Children. Education Survey 1*, HMSO, 1967, p.45.
4　DES. *Integrating handicapped children*, HMSO, 1976, p.16.
5　DES. *Units for Partially Hearing Children. Education Survey 1*, HMSO, 1967, p.32.
6　National Youth Employment Council. *Report on the Youth Employment Service*, 1950/53, p.9.

Chapter 8

Pre-lingually deaf adults

For most adults who became deaf before the acquisition of speech and language, habilitation involves interpretation and meeting their vocational, spiritual and recreational needs.

Interpretation

The difficulties that a pre-lingually deaf child has to overcome in acquiring speech and language have been described in an earlier chapter. The educational goal of the oral system as taught in schools for the deaf has been defined as 'to enable the deaf child to achieve fluent, audible, rhythmic and intelligible speech in order that other people may understand it'.[1] Where an adequate command of language has been attained and speech and speech-reading developed to a high degree of efficiency, the integration of a deaf person into normal society is claimed to be possible. A consequence of such integration is that 'the world of persons, ideas and experiences open to him (the deaf child) is richer and more varied than the restricted world of the deaf. He does not acquire the sense of being different that affects the deaf who are cut off from normal communication with their fellows.'

Not all pre-lingually deaf pupils succeed in mastering the oral system to the extent that their command of speech and speech-reading is adequate for social competency. Studies by Conrad[2] and Denmark[3] have shown that only a minority of pupils on leaving school have attained a high level of oral proficiency. In the Denmark study, the rating by parents of the post-school speech skills of 43 profoundly deaf and 32 partially hearing adolescents resulted in Table 8.1.

77

Table 8.1 Parents' rating of adolescents' post-school speech skills (Denmark)

Talking to hearing people	Profoundly deaf		Partially hearing	
	No.	%	No.	%
Easily	4	9	12	37.5
Some difficulty	23	54	13	40.5
Extreme difficulty	8	19	7	22
Unable unless hearing person used to deaf	6	14	0	0
Totally unable	1	2	0	0
No response	1	2	0	0
Total	43	100	32	100

Only 9 per cent of the profoundly deaf school leavers have speech and speech-reading skills which are sufficient to enable them to talk easily with hearing people; 16 per cent are totally unable to do so. The same study showed a clear preference by both groups for manual methods of communication when the respondents were speaking both to hearing people and deaf peers.

For deaf persons who have either failed to achieve socially adequate communication through the oral system or who have abandoned the effort to comprehend and participate in the non-deaf milieu, situations will arise where the use of an interpreter is essential. It is no exaggeration to claim that every aspect of welfare for deaf persons using manual communication methods involves interpretation.

Basically interpretation involves two elements: the transposing of the sound of words into a visible form and paraphrasing, explaining or simplifying the words used so that the meaning intended by the speaker is understood by the deaf person.

Two warnings relating to interpretation are important. Firstly, the persons with a merely superficial knowledge of finger-spelling and signing are unsuitable as interpreters. Secondly, interpretation involves more than the mere converting of words into sound and requires a knowledge of the psychology and outlook of deaf persons both individually and in the group. An example, furnished by a social worker for the deaf illustrates the incompetency of untrained persons to undertake interpretation.

Some time ago I had to interpret for four young men who had been arrested for shoplifting. They told me they had been put in the dock and someone came forward and did a lot of finger-spelling which they could not understand. They said that they stood there like a lot of fools but apparently neither the magistrate nor the police realised that they understood nothing. It is this that makes us realise that a superficial knowledge of the deaf is worse than useless.

The Home Office has agreed with the Association of Directors of Social Services and the RNID that where deaf persons are involved in court proceedings, chief officers of police should contact the local Director of Social Services or, in case of difficulty, the RNID, to request that an interpreter should be provided. Similar assistance should be provided for deaf and deaf-blind persons appearing before Mental Review Tribunals.

Few people with normal hearing, however, are able to communicate by manual methods. The need to increase the number and standard of interpreters received a stimulus in 1977 when the BDA was given funding by the DHSS for a project to develop communication skills and establish a Register of Interpreters. *The Council for the Advancement of Communication with Deaf Persons* (CACDP) was founded in 1980. The main aims of the CACDP are:

1   To promote training and conduct examinations in communication skills.
2   To maintain and administer a Register of Interpreters.
3   To encourage research and collate information relevant to the above aims.

When the Council's system of training and assessment in sign communication is fully developed, certificates will be awarded for competence at elementary, intermediate and final levels. Completion of the final level and a post-qualifying year in which applicants must satisfy the Council's examiners of their interpreting ability in specific settings are required before admission to the Register of Interpreters.

Other needs of adult deaf persons

Deaf persons have the same basic needs and rights as other citizens but their handicap often makes it difficult for such needs to be satisfied or their rights to be fully exercised. In this book only a brief treatment is possible of the needs for personal service, spiritual ministration, employment, and recreation, and a brief discussion of the special problems encountered by deaf persons with mental illness and the deaf-blind.

Personal services

Normally most deaf people manage their personal, domestic and working lives as well as other members of the community. In times of crisis, however, they need the help of someone who can communicate fully with them. Usually this will be a social worker for the deaf either employed directly by a local authority or a voluntary society providing services for the deaf on behalf of an authority under an agency agreement. The effectiveness of the personal service provided depends largely on the competency of a social worker in communication skills. Where such skills are inadequate it is not unusual for deaf persons preferring manual methods of communication to seek help outside the area in which they live. Problems may also arise when only one social worker in an area can communicate with the deaf. Burton[4] has emphasised the affront to the dignity of deaf persons who, in such circumstances, have to be accompanied on visits to a doctor or hospital by an interpreter of the opposite sex. When the Register of Interpreters, referred to earlier, is fully operative, the range of safeguards, choice and opportunities for deaf persons will be considerably extended. In providing personal services for deaf clients social workers may co-operate with other specialists such as psychiatric social workers or on occasion act as agents providing the services normally provided by probation or disablement resettlement officers. Because of their communication skills they will be the link between deaf persons, their families, neighbours and to mention but a few others, employers, the clergy, trade union officials, teachers and the staffs of central and local government departments concerned with health, housing, employment and social security.

Stress on the communication function should not, however, overshadow the direct counselling and other roles of social workers with deaf persons. Among such roles are those of adviser and confidant particularly regarding problems arising from sickness, marriage, bereavement and similar crises; of provider, in making available resources available from the social workers' own and other agencies and of advocate in presenting the claims of the deaf person for such resources to the right quarter. In fulfilling all these roles social workers for the deaf must try to develop the capacity for independent action on the part of those who seek their assistance. They must always be conscious, however,

that if they cannot find time to listen to a deaf client there may be no-one else able to do so. The pre-lingually deaf client cannot take his minor troubles to a neighbour . . . and he may be without a family living near or not wishing to contact the family. During a period of severe illness or at times of bereavement, he may need both factual information and intensive social work help.[5]

Spiritual ministration

Because the numbers of pre-lingually deaf persons in any locality is relatively small, any denominationalism in spiritual work other than the broad divisions of Protestant and Roman Catholic is impracticable. Anglican work for the deaf is co-ordinated by the *General Synod Council for the Deaf* (GSCD). While the chief object of the GSCD is to help those born severely or totally deaf, it is anxious to help those with any hearing impairment. A forum for representatives from each of the 75 churches for the deaf in the country is provided by the *National Deaf Church Conference,* which endeavours to provide a link between autonomous worshipping communities. The examinations of the *Chaplains to the Deaf Examinations Board* are open to both ordained priests and ministers and lay ministers of all denominations whether working among deaf people in a full- or part-time capacity.

Roman Catholic work for the deaf is under the auspices of the *Association for the Roman Catholic Deaf in Great Britain and Ireland.*

Spiritual work provides many opportunities for the participation of deaf persons. *The Ecumenical Council of Christian Workers with the Deaf* is closely involved in the provision of training facilities for deaf lay helpers and arranges courses designed to enable deaf people to take a leadership role within their communities. In some churches there are deaf choirs which endeavour to sing hymns in unison. It has been stated that 'Sign and gesture language can be refined and beautified till it becomes not only the easiest form of utterance for the deaf but all they can ever realise of poetry and music'.[6]

Employment

In seeking to obtain and retain employment a deaf person may be assisted by several services provided by the *Employment Service Agency* of the *Manpower Services Commission* (MSC).

Registration on the Disabled Persons' Register

Registration, which is voluntary, may be granted for any period from one to ten years or until the date of retirement depending on the nature of the disablement. Some schools for the deaf ensure that all their leavers register. The BDA also advises its members to register.

Assistance from the disablement resettlement officer (DRO)

The DRO is trained to help disabled people to find jobs they can do well and with satisfaction. At the same time the DRO will ensure that disabled persons make the best use of the services that are open to them. In assessing the suitability of jobs for deaf persons a DRO should take three main factors into consideration.

Firstly, is there anything about the job which makes it especially suitable for a deaf employee? A person who is not distracted by noise, for example, is likely to be better able to concentrate than a hearing worker providing the noise level is not so great that the vibrations are painful. It is possible that for some jobs 'deafness' could be a desirable factor in a job description.

Secondly, to what extent is hearing and speech required by the job? According to a survey undertaken by the Manpower Administration of the US Department of Labor of some 13,000 jobs, hearing and speech are not required by approximately 80 per cent of those listed. The Labor Department analyses consider such factors as the effect on production and safety, the need to convey oral information to the public, to give and receive spoken instructions and to make fine discrimination between sounds.

Thirdly, what situational factors relating to the job are of significance to a deaf person? At least five situational factors can be identified:

1 The complexity of job instruction and how instruction can be conveyed; whether the job can be learned mainly by observation.
2 The character of supervision. Deaf persons learn more easily from a patient, person-centred supervisor than one who resents the loss of production entailed in instructing a new employee who is deaf.
3 Whether hearing workers are likely to be helpful and sympathetic to a deaf colleague.

4   Whether warning signals are exclusively auditory. This is particularly important if a deaf person is to work in an isolated location.

5   Whether adjustments to the job or work routine are possible in order to make it suitable for a deaf person.

The main objections by employers to taking on a deaf person will probably refer to communication difficulties, accident proneness, failure to hear warning signals, inability to use the telephone and possible objections to working with a deaf person by hearing members of the work-force. Against these objections a DRO can state the positive qualities of deaf workers. These include the following:

1   Deaf workers tend to appreciate employment opportunities more than their hearing counterparts.

2   They may be more conscientious.

3   They are less likely to be distracted by conversation or other disturbances than hearing employees.

4   Especially with work of a routine nature their job perform-ance is not inferior to workers with normal hearing.

5   The attendance record of deaf workers is generally good.

It is, however, important to be honest with a prospective employer about the capabilities of a potential deaf employee since an unsatisfactory placement may prejudice other oppor-tunities for deaf workers with that undertaking. Full information should therefore be made available to an employer regarding the severity of the applicant's deafness, communication methods used, educational and any previous work record, vocational training and personality factors.

There is evidence that the best results in placing pre-lingually deaf persons in employment are obtained when the DRO works closely with a social worker (employed either by a local authority or a voluntary society) who possesses a high level of competency in interpretation. The publication *Employing Someone who is Deaf or Hard of Hearing* issued by the Employment Service Agency states specifically that:

Interpreters who have acquired special skills in communicating with deaf people – using finger-spelling, signs or speech – are available throughout the country to help with the interviewing of deaf people for jobs. Some are qualified social workers who have expert knowledge of the problems of deafness and of the capabilities of deaf people.

Interpretation in connection with placement work, however,

is not confined to facilitating communication at the engagement interview. At the commencement of employment the social
worker for the deaf may assist in interpreting instructions
relative to the performance of duties to deaf persons who
experience difficulty in comprehension. The writer recalls one
welfare officer for the deaf, employed by a voluntary society,
who enabled two deaf men to move from unskilled work to
employment as skilled weavers. The welfare officer attended the
factory and was trained as a weaver himself. At the same time he
instructed the two deaf learners in the processes involved. The
social worker may also assist the deaf person to settle into
employment and help the employer with any problems arising
from the engagement of a deaf employee. Because he is a non-
hearing person in a hearing environment the need to adjust lies
primarily with the deaf worker rather than with his hearing
associates. Imperfect comprehension of instructions, for
example, may cause annoyance both on the part of a hearing
supervisor and the deaf person who may claim that he is being
exploited or ridiculed. Thus, the social worker may play an
important role not only in helping a deaf person to obtain
employment but also in retaining it.

Other services

Deaf persons may also avail themselves of the range of services
for disabled persons and their employers provided by the
Manpower Services Commission. Incentives to employers
include grants under the Job Introduction Scheme in respect of
disabled persons who are taken on for a trial period. Employers
may also receive grants of up to £6,000 towards adaptation of
their premises and equipment required to enable them to
employ or retain a disabled person. Special aids including
telephone aids, earpiece amplifiers and loudspeaking telephones may be bought and issued on free permanent loan to
enable a disabled person to keep employment.

Deaf persons are also eligible to participate in training
schemes arranged by the *Training Services Division* of the MSC.
These include Training Opportunities courses at skills centres,
technical and commercial colleges and the *Individual Training
Throughout with an Employer* (ITTWE) scheme. Residential
training is offered at four residential colleges and professional
training is available to those with the necessary educational

background and ability who wish to train for a professional career including a university degree. Details of all these facilities can be obtained from the DRO.

A study by Kyle and Allsop[7] of 227 persons with a profound hearing loss resident in the county of Avon reported that only 2 per cent of those in employment who were interviewed had a supervisory role; 81 per cent stated that they were never involved in planning their work and only 12 per cent anticipated promotion within the next two years. The statement, frequently made, that deaf persons are underemployed therefore seems well justified. A fact sheet[8] issued by the MSC warns employers against assuming that disabled employees prefer not to take on more responsibility, work under pressure, change their jobs or lack ambition because they are disabled. This warning is not without relevance to deaf persons.

Recreation and leisure

Deaf persons may experience considerable isolation both at home and work due to the inability of most hearing people to converse by signs and finger-spelling. In such circumstances an intense hunger for social life and companionship may impel them to seek the company of others using similar communication methods at a club or centre for deaf persons; where no specific centre is available, the deaf may congregate at informal meeting places such as a particular public house. Rodda[9] found that the degree of hearing loss, its age of onset and attendance at a special school were the principal factors influencing whether a deaf person would attend a deaf club. Clubs for the deaf were more attractive to persons with a profound pre-lingual loss.

Social clubs for deaf persons may provide a range of indoor and outdoor activities. Apart from sports and games these include bingo, dancing, drama groups, holidays and outings and watching television. The promotion of amateur sports and games among the deaf of Great Britain is undertaken by the British Deaf Sports Council (BDSC). Working through some 120 clubs and 11 regional councils the BDSC organises sports and games locally, regionally, nationally and internationally. The range of indoor and outdoor sports promoted includes: billiards/ snooker, chess, darts, squash, table tennis, angling, athletics, badminton, bowling, cricket, cycling, football, netball, skiing, swimming, tennis and waterskiing. Through its affiliation with the International Committee for Deaf Sports which has some 60 member countries, the BDSC sends British representatives every four years to European and World Games in which approximately 8,000 deaf athletes compete.

Jones,[10] however, reports that activities were hardly mentioned by any of his respondents who gave 'company' and 'signs' as the main reasons for their attendance at social centres for the deaf. The importance of conversation to the deaf has been well expressed by a former welfare officer for the deaf then working in a rural area:

The deaf read the newspapers at home but they cannot say to their relatives: 'Have you seen the news?' or 'What do you think of this?' They save it up until they come to the club and then discuss the news or ask about the things they have seen in the papers . . . often when asked if they would like to play games, they say: 'I can play billiards or darts at the village institute or at home with hearing friends but I have no one to sign to at home. I don't pay fares to come and play games. I want to talk.'

As another welfare officer observed to the writer, 'Conversation is usually gossip, but to the deaf, gossip is the essence of life.'

Deaf persons with mental illness

The danger of using inappropriate psychological tests to assess the intelligence or personality of pre-lingually deaf persons was stressed in Chapter 5. When a psychiatrist is unable to communicate by signs and finger-spelling with a deaf person who has unintelligible speech and a poor command of language, there is a danger of wrong diagnosis or confusion with mental retardation. One example from many quoted by Denmark, a consultant psychiatrist, who acquired facility in manual communication as a child at the residential school for the deaf of which his father was headmaster, is given below:

C M, a 25 year old man, had been remanded to prison having been charged with assault. He suffers from pre-lingual deafness, is without speech and his language is limited. He had become aggressive when asked to leave the house of his girlfriend's mother, who did not wish his association with her daughter to continue. In referring him the prison doctor had written . . . 'He may be schizophrenic, mentally defective, or anything.' Using manual communication methods C M was able to give a good account of himself, explaining that he resented being pushed out of his girlfriend's home without, he felt, good cause. He became very angry when he could not understand what was being said and because he could not conduct his own thoughts and feelings. When examined using manual communication methods there was no evidence of any material psychiatric abnormality and, using non-verbal psychological tests, he achieved a pro rated IQ of 116.[11]

Denmark was mainly responsible for the establishment in 1968 of a psychiatric unit for the deaf at Whittingham Hospital, near Preston, which was the first centre of its kind in the UK. Out-patient clinics are held in Manchester and London and patients requiring further investigation or in-patient treatment are admitted to the Whittingham unit. Psychiatric services for the deaf are also available at Richardson House, Blackburn for the rehabilitation of young persons with a history of psychiatric problems, Springfield Hospital, London SW17 and the Gartnavel Royal and Leverndale Hospitals in Glasgow. The RNID also has a residential centre at Poolemead, Bristol.

In addition to the assessment and treatment of patients, the Whittingham Hospital provides training courses for nurses, social workers and others who require a knowledge of total communication methods and the psychological and psychiatric aspects of deafness. In assisting a psychiatrist a social worker for the deaf with a good skill in total communication may act as interpreter, adviser and protector. As interpreter he may facilitate the rapidity and accuracy of communication between the psychiatrist and the deaf person. As adviser he can often provide, from his personal knowledge of a deaf individual, particulars relative to such matters as the family background and social life which can assist the psychiatrist in his understanding and diagnosis of the case. As protector he can ensure that slow comprehension and imperfect speech are not by themselves regarded as indicating mental retardation or disorder.

The RNID has repeatedly advocated that an interpreter should be present in all cases where the compulsory detention of deaf persons believed to be suffering from mental illness is contemplated. By visitation a social worker for the deaf can help to alleviate the isolation experienced by hearing impaired persons who are in-patients in mental hospitals. After discharge the social worker can assist with the family, social and occupational

rehabilitation of the deaf person and also, by careful observation, ensure that any signs of the recurrence of mental illness
do not go undetected.

The deaf-blind

A deaf-blind person may be described as one who by reason of
impaired hearing and vision is forced to rely considerably or
entirely on the remaining senses of touch, taste and smell with
touch normally playing the major role. Apart from the relatively
few cases in which a person is congenitally deaf and blind, a
somewhat arbitary distinction may be made between the deaf-
blind and blind-deaf according to whether deafness or blindness
was the primary impairment. This distinction is important since
the psycho-social development and habilitation of the individual will be influenced according to whether blindness or
deafness occurred first. As Verstrate[12] points out:

Those who have once had vision can relate to colour, to visual images
that we can convey verbally. They will, in most cases, respond to the
printing of letters on the palm. Those who have at one time heard may be
able to relate to auditory references – sounds of everyday living,
references to music with which they have been familiar, or any of those
stimuli which once had association for the now non-hearing person.

An important aspect of the habilitation of deaf-blind persons
is therefore the utilisation and conservation of residual auditory
and visual abilities. Numerically the incidence of deaf-blindness
is small. In 1979 the number of persons on the register of the
blind who were reported to have the additional handicap of
deafness was:

Age	Number
0–15	32
16–64	343
65 and over	1,570

These statistics were certainly an understatement and it is
probable that the total number of blind persons in the UK who
additionally are deaf with or without speech or hard of hearing
will be about 5,000. Only very few of the total blind population
are deaf-blind to such a degree that they cannot be helped by any
hearing aid. The incidence of deaf-blindness clearly rises steeply
with age. The small numbers, however, conceal a great deal of
loneliness and frustration.

As with all cases of hearing impairment the main difficulty to be overcome is that of auditory communication but this is complicated by the lack of vision. Apart from communication through an interpreter, use can be made of the special manual alphabet which comprises a series of signs made on the left hand of the deaf-blind person. This method of communication is described in a leaflet, *How to talk to a Person who is Deaf and Blind*, which is issued free by the Southern and Western Regional Association for the Blind. Another method of communication is to trace block capitals with the index finger with the pattern of strokes used in writing on the deaf-blind person's left hand. All deaf-blind people should of course be given the opportunity of learning to use Braille. For those who have lost their delicacy of touch or who find the Braille notation too difficult the simpler Moon type may be taught. Klemz[13] has rightly stated that 'For those who cannot hear radio and talking books Braille and Moon are the only links with the world of culture and current affairs.' The Royal National Institute for the Blind (RNIB) will provide a list of special aids for deaf-blind persons; some of the special aids for the deaf described in Chapter 10 may also be applicable.

Educational provision for deaf-blind children is, from a geographical standpoint, unevenly spread. The largest centre is Pathways, Andover Hall, Shrewsbury, where there are about 30 deaf-blind children in an all-age, special department of a school for multiply-handicapped, blind pupils. Other residential units are located at the Royal Victoria School for the Blind, Newcastle-on-Tyne and the Royal School for the Deaf, Margate. In London four schools for children with special educational needs have deaf-blind pupils integrated into normal groups and a number of other units for multiply-handicapped children also cater for those who are deaf and blind. The National Association for Deaf-Blind and Rubella Handicapped has a Residential and Further Education Centre for young deaf-blind adults at The Manor House, Market Deeping, Lincolnshire. The RNID also has a centre for deaf-blind young people aged 16+ who, while probably less able than those at Market Deeping, can still benefit from social and/or occupational training.

A special committee of the RNIB is concerned with the deaf-blind. The Royal Association in Aid of the Deaf and Dumb has a specialist worker for deaf-blind people. The National Deaf-Blind Helpers' League brings deaf-blind persons together through regional group activities and rallies and publishes a quarterly magazine, *The Rainbow,* in Braille, Moon and print. This organisation also provides deaf-blind people capable of running their own homes with private, self-contained flats and has a small guest house and short-stay centre in Peterborough. Mention should also be made of the Deaf-Blind Fellowship which amongst other activities organises holidays.

References

1 Ewing, I. R. and A. W. G. *Opportunity and the Deaf Child,* University of London Press Limited, 1950, Ch. 14, p.159.
2 Conrad, R. *The Deaf School Child,* Harper and Row, 1979.
3 Denmark and others. *A Word in Deaf Ears – A Study of Communication and Behaviour in a Sample of Deaf Adolescents undertaken by the Department of Psychiatry for the Deaf, Whittingham Hospital and the Social Research Branch,* DHSS, 1979.
4 Burton, D. 'Services for Deaf Persons in the New Social Services Departments', Paper given to the biennial conference of the RNID, 1972.
5 National Council of Social Workers with the Deaf. Evidence given to the National Institute for Social Work, April 1981.
6 Quoted in Mackenzie, A. C. 'Methods of Conducting Divine Service for the Deaf', Typewritten pamphlet (undated) in the RNID Library.
7 Kyle and Allsop. *Deaf People and the Community,* Report to the Nuffield Foundation, School of Education Research Unit, University of Bristol, 1981.
8 MSC. *Employers Factsheet No.6,* January 1982.
9 Rodda, M. *The Hearing Impaired School Leaver,* University of London Press, 1970, p.159.
10 Jones, K. D. 'The Adult Deaf Population of South Humberside'. Unpublished M Phil. thesis, University of Nottingham, 1983, p.110.
11 Denmark, J. C. 'Early Profound Deafness and Mental Retardation', *British Journal of Mental Subnormality,* Vol. XXIV, Part 2, No. 47, Dec. 1978.
12 Verstrate, Donna. *Social Group Work with Deaf-Blind Adults.* American Foundation for the Blind, New York, 1959, p.9.
13 Klemz, Astrid. *Blindness and Partial Sight,* Woodhead-Faulkner, 1977, p.122.

Chapter 9

Deafened and hard of hearing adults

A distinction between 'disability' and 'handicap' was made in Chapter 1 and some limitations of speech audiometry were briefly mentioned in Chapter 4. Particularly with deafened and hard of hearing persons it is important to recognise that the severity of hearing loss as indicated by pure-tone and speech audiometry provides only limited information of the extent to which a given individual is handicapped. For purposes of habilitation or rehabilitation it is necessary to supplement audiometric assessments by other procedures designed to elicit further data regarding the ability of the individual to overcome, as far as possible, the limitations imposed by hearing impairment.

Evaluating hearing handicap

The degree to which a disability constitutes a handicap is influenced by many factors. Age, intelligence, personality, vocational aspirations, the occupational importance of auditory communication, aptitude for speech-reading, family support and the attitudes to hearing loss of work and other associates are some variables to be considered in determining the extent to which handicap can be mitigated. A number of tests have been devised to obtain data regarding attitudes to hearing impairment, communication performance in various environments and the problems that an individual encounters as a result of hearing loss. Two of the earliest tests were the *Bronfenbrenner Hearing Attitude Scale* and the *Social Adequacy Index*. The Bronfenbrenner Scale described in the *Psychology of Deafness* by

91

Edna S. Levine[1] was developed between 1944 and 1945 for use with a rehabilitation programme for members of the US forces who had sustained hearing impairments ranging from minimal to severe in World War II. The purpose of the test was to evaluate the attitudes of a person to hearing loss in relation to the following: self-appraisal; depression; over-optimism; tension; reaction to rehabilitation; job worry; sensitivity; cover-up; withdrawal and eccentric reactions. Respondents were asked to encircle 'Agree' or 'Disagree' to each of 100 simply-worded statements describing possible reactions to situations encountered as a result of hearing loss. Two typical statements are:

Being hard of hearing would stop me
from taking a job where I have to be boss   Agree   Disagree
I won't wear a hearing aid under any
conditions   Agree   Disagree

This scale, suitably modified, is still useful as an interview guide.

The Social Adequacy Index[2] measured the relationship between the percentage of words correctly understood, known as the articulation score, and the speech reception threshold or intensity level at which words reach the ear of the listener. The Index was therefore a single number that indicated how well a person heard speech under average everyday conditions. It relied however on speech audiometry and did not allow for individual differences encountered across a wide range of communication situations.

An attempt to describe all the various non-audiometric tests of hearing handicap is impossible within the scope of this book and the interested reader is referred to Alpiner, J. (Ed.). *Handbook of Adult Rehabilitation Audiology*[3] which contains examples of numerous tests. Three tests of special importance may be briefly described: these are the *Hearing Handicap Scale*, the *Social Hearing Handicap Index* and *The Hearing Measurement Scale*. The questionnaires used for these tests are shown in Appendix 2.

The Hearing Handicap Scale (HHS)

HHS is a self-assessment procedure developed in America by High, Fairbanks and Glorig in 1964.[4] Handicap in this context is defined as 'any disadvantage in the activities of everyday living which derives from hearing impairment'. Two parallel forms each containing 20 items are presented. The items relate to ordinary experiences likely to have been encountered by most persons living in an urban environment. The majority of items describe experiences involving speech communication; the remainder deal with hearing for background noise and warning signals. Respondents are required to indicate on a scale of relative frequency ranging from 'almost always' to 'almost never' how often difficulty has been experienced with the auditory event specified in the item. The disadvantages of the HHS, recognised by its authors, are that answers may easily be falsified and that it provides no information on the psychological, vocational and other consequences of hearing loss.

The Social Hearing Handicap Index (SHHI)

This is also a self-assessment procedure developed in Denmark as a derivative of the HHS by Ewertsen and Birk-Nielsen in 1973.[5] The Index was developed to measure psychological, vocational and family aspects of hearing loss not obtainable from audiometric testing. The questionnaire of 21 items relates to conversation in quiet and noisy environments, group situations, telephone usage and ability to understand speech from radio or television. Respondents are required to provide 'Yes' or 'No' answers. A respondent with a hearing handicap will have to answer 'No' and 'Yes' in 10 and 11 cases respectively. If the respondent has not encountered the situation posed by the question, the answer 'I do not know' is required, while if unsure, the probable answer is enclosed in brackets, (Yes) or (No). A clear 'Yes' or 'No' answer scores 2 points. If in brackets, the score is 1 and 'Do not know' is 0. The handicap score (h) lies between 0 and 42, but to adjust it to the decimal system the following social handicap index (SHI) is used:

$$SHI = \frac{h}{42} \times 100$$

This gives an index scale from 0 to 100 where 0 means no handicap and 100 a maximum handicap. The authors did not find any relationship between the duration of the hearing impairment and the degree of social handicap or between age and handicap but found that speech-reading capacity had a definite influence on the hearing handicapped.

The Hearing Measurement Scale

The aim in devising this inventory[6] was to devise and develop a scale, in the form of a standard interview, for the measurement of auditory disability in those with cochlear sensorineural disorder due to noise exposure. Hearing handicap is defined as 'the response of the sufferer to hearing loss and includes the emotional reaction to situations in which hearing difficulty occurs plus the opinion of the individual about his hearing'.

This scale, which is the only one to have been standardised in the UK and is being increasingly used for research and rehabilitation, comprises a 42-item test divided into seven sections:

1   Hearing for speech.
2   Hearing for non-speech sound.
3   Localisation.
4   Emotional response.
5   Speech distortion.
6   Tinnitus.
7   Personal opinion.

Each section has a weighted score with a possible maximum overall totalling 226. The test is designed to be administered in an interview situation. To score and administer the test a manual of instructions obtainable only from the principal author is required. The main disadvantage is the interview time required (10–40 minutes) but a modified paper and pencil test has been devised. Though developed for adults with cochlear sensorineural disorders the test has been found equally useful for assessing handicap due to hearing impairment from other causes.

Open-ended questionnaires

While open-ended questionnaires may provide both more and more reliable information, they have not been extensively used because of the difficulty of scoring the responses. One example of the use of an open-ended questionnaire designed to ascertain what hearing impaired people themselves considered to be the main problems arising from their disability is described by Barcham and Stephens.[7] The questionnaire, sent out with the appointment letters to all patients attending the Department of Auditory Rehabilitation of the Royal National Throat, Nose and

Ear Hospital, London for the first time was worded as follows:

Please make a list of the difficulties which you have as a result of your hearing loss. List them in order of importance, starting with the biggest difficulties. Write down as many as you can think of.

As the responses were listed in decreasing order of importance the authors gave the first problem mentioned a score of 5 and the second, third and fourth problems scores of 4, 3 and 2 respectively. The fifth and all subsequent problems were scored 1. From the first 500 replies received, the authors identified certain major groupings of problems such as conversational difficulties, environmental sounds, medical responses and psychological problems. These are shown in Tables 9.1 – 9.5. Table 9.1 includes all the major problems, i.e. those mentioned by more than 100 people. Table 9.2 shows secondary problems mentioned by more than 50 but less than 100 people. Table 9.3 covers problems stated by 10 or more, but less than 50 respondents. Medical responses and psychological problems are reported in Tables 9.4 and 9.5 respectively.

Table 9.1 Major response categories

Difficulty	Number of respondents	Percentage of total respondents	Mean weighting of responses
TV Radio	241	48	2.9
General conversation	170	34	4.2
Doorbell	119	24	2.6
Group conversation	114	23	3.9
Speech in noise	114	23	3.5
Telephone bell	102	20	2.7
Meetings	102	20	2.9

The authors point out that an open-ended questionnaire can be useful in identifying possible areas for further investigation; e.g. employment problems, counselling with regard to hearing and environmental aids and assessing the benefit a person has received from the rehabilitation service by comparing replies completed six or nine months after a hearing aid has been fitted with those completed before rehabilitation began.

Special problems of deafened and hard of hearing persons

Apart from communication and the psychological aspects of

hearing loss, a deafened or hard of hearing person may encounter problems in four areas: tinnitus, speech conservation, employment, family attitudes.

Tinnitus

Tinnitus, from the Latin verb *tinnire*, 'to ring', has been defined as the sensation of sound in the absence of an external stimulus. Head noises accompany almost all forms of hearing impairment

Table 9.2 Secondary response categories

Difficulty	Number of respondents	Percentage of total respondents	Mean weighting
Speech from one direction	97	19	2.9
Telephone conversation	97	19	2.7
Quiet voices	83	17	2.7
Hearing without lip-reading	76	15	3.2
Embarrassment	69	14	2.9
Employment problems	63	12	4.3
Conversation with strangers	62	12	4.3
Discrimination of words, warning signals, alarms, sirens, horns, traffic, etc.	53	11	2.9

Table 9.3 Minor response categories

Difficulty	Number of respondents	Percentage of total respondents	Mean weighting
Hearing when called	49	10	2.7
Theatre/cinema	48	10	2.9
Hearing children speak	33	7	3.0
Depression, strain	30	6	2.3
Localisation	30	6	3.1
Domestic warning noises: door shutting, kettle boiling, etc	27	5	2.7
Loneliness	26	5	3.0
Music	23	4	2.9
Hearing speech from a distance	22	4	3.0
One to one conversation	20	4	4.1
Hearing a clock or watch	18	4	1.6
Not hearing environmental noises	18	4	1.8
Public address systems	15	3	1.9
Family strain	14	3	2.1
Lack of confidence	10	2	4.1
Foreign accents, dialects, etc.	10	2	3.3

Table 9.4 Medical responses

Difficulty	Number of respondents	Percentage of total respondents	Mean weighting
Tinnitus	40	8	3.8
Fluctuant hearing loss	19	4	2.7
Vertigo	10	2	1.9
Sinusitis	10	2	2.0
Recruitment	10	2	2.7
Pressure in the ears	10	2	3.0

Table 9.5 Psychological problems

Difficulty	Number of respondents	Percentage of total respondents	Mean weighting
Embarrassment	69	14	2.9
Nervous strain	30	6	2.3
Loneliness	26	5	3.0
Family strain	14	3	2.1
Lack of confidence	10	2	4.1

and may range from 'mild' to 'severe'. An estimated 300,000 people in the UK find that tinnitus makes life almost unbearable. A distinction may be made between subjective and objective tinnitus. With subjective tinnitus the head noises are audible only to the person affected. In objective tinnitus, which is less common, and usually has little to do with hearing, the noises are also audible to others. A further distinction is between simple tinnitus and auditory hallucination. With the former the sounds heard are simple monotones variously described as 'ringing', 'throbbing' etc. The latter refers to the sensation of hearing more complex and cacophonous sounds often described as 'guns going off', 'a peal of bells' or 'a devil's orchestra.

The causes of tinnitus are as diverse as those of hearing impairment. Three common causes are obstructions to sound conduction, pathological alterations in the cells of the cochlear sensory system and the physical distortion of the cochlear sensory system. Tinnitus may be due to such conductive causes as wax, otitis-media or otosclerosis arising in the outer or middle ears. Pathological changes may be induced by noise or drugs. Physical distortion of the cochlear system is usually responsible for the tinnitus that accompanies Ménière's Disease.

The treatment of tinnitus clearly depends on its cause. Tinnitus due to conductive obstruction often disappears if the predisposing cause is successfully treated. The restoration of hearing by middle ear surgery, for example, is often accompanied by the disappearance of tinnitus. In most cases, however, tinnitus is intractable and it is relief rather than cure that is the object of treatment. Drugs such as Lignocaine, Praxilene and Amylobarbitone may alleviate the condition.

For the majority of tinnitus sufferers a 'tinnitus masker' may be the most effective treatment. A masker is essentially a device by which a band of white noise is fed, usually to the affected ear, thereby making the tinnitus either inaudible or less troublesome. Maskers can be incorporated in either behind-the-ear or in-the-ear aids. Bedside maskers are also available to help sufferers to mask the tinnitus and thereby sleep better. Theoretically, maskers are obtainable from the NHS and enquiries should be made through the ENT department of the local hospital. Maskers may also be bought through private hearing aid dispensers. The RNID recommends that, as a masker is not always successful, it should initially be used for a trial period before the purchase is completed. Wood[8] reports that in approximately 50 per cent of cases the phenomenon called 'residual inhibition' occurs. Residual inhibition means that following a period of masker use the tinnitus is wholly or partly suppressed for a period of time. 'In a small proportion, about 4 per cent, residual inhibition occurs and the masker needs only to be used for short periods, say five or ten minutes at various times of the day to produce total suppression.'

As an alternative to a masker some tinnitus sufferers find temporary relief by turning up their hearing aids to secure maximum amplification thereby blotting out the head noises.

Apart from drugs and maskers a person with tinnitus has to 'learn to live with it'. Given courage and a constructive attitude it is possible to become at least partially adjusted to tinnitus. Some advice given by C. H. Mardell, a former Secretary of the British Association of the Hard of Hearing, himself a tinnitus sufferer for many years, is helpful:

The best way to treat tinnitus is the same as one treats the club bore. You accept you must listen to him and you do so with the best grace you can. So if the head noises are unduly loud, to listen to them makes them as acceptable as much as anything can; and trying to put them out of one's mind, being impossible, is a useless waste of emotion. The practice of listening to them does work and I would commend it as the only thing one can do to help, i.e. after a short while your mind wanders off them.

The British Tinnitus Association was launched by the RNID in 1979. The primary aims of the Association are to spread knowledge about tinnitus and the help or treatments available, amongst the medical profession and amongst sufferers; to encourage the formation of self-help groups; to raise money for research; and to act as a pressure group for greater Government support. The Association now has several thousand members and about 70 local groups spread throughout the UK. A most informative quarterly newsletter is circulated to members.

Speech conservation

Speech conservation is an essential aspect of auditory rehabilitation, especially where the hearing loss is so severe that the person affected has difficulty in monitoring his speech and voice due to the absence of auditory feedback. Even a relatively mild loss will affect the pitch of speech as is evidenced by the soft, low speech of a person with a conductive impairment and the relatively loud speech of someone with a sensorineural loss. The rate at which speech will deteriorate will depend on a number of factors including the type and severity of hearing loss, the time of onset, the rate of deterioration of hearing loss, the extent to which residual hearing can be utilised and the length of time between the need for speech conservation and its actual provision.

Speech conservation is the province of the speech therapist who will have obtained a qualification recognised by the College of Speech Therapists. After qualification, most speech therapists function within the National Health Service.

Work with hearing impaired children and adults is one of the more recent specialisations within the field of speech therapy. Irlam, Wechsler and Parker[9] point out that the involvement of speech therapists in audiological services usually takes two main forms, namely those who work in general assessment clinics such as those found in hospitals and those who, as members of a specialist otological/audiological team, have 'responsibility for communication, language and speech assessment in addition to more general audiological evaluation'. In both cases close co-operation with other specialists such as otologists, audiologists and teachers of the deaf is essential.

With adventitiously deafened or hard of hearing persons the aim of the speech therapist is to preserve speech production skills that are in danger of deteriorating. Brown[10] suggests that regulation of voice quality, pitch and the rate of speaking are the first problems to which attention may need to be directed followed by those relating to articulation. There is evidence that the procedures used lead not only to improved speech but also exercise a significant reinforcing effect on speech-reading proficiency and auditory training and increased confidence on the part of a severely hearing impaired person in communication situations.

The first step in speech conservation is the evaluation of the individual's speech both to ascertain what remedial action is required and to compare the results of speech therapy. Such evaluation should relate to the aesthetic quality and intelligibility of speech and the identification of auditory defects. The aesthetic quality of speech relates to such aspects as voice quality, pitch, intonation, loudness, rate of speaking and rhythm. Thus, the voice quality of a person with a profound loss may be characterised by little, if any, variation in pitch and the inability to control such variations that occur. Intelligibility relates to the extent to which speech can be understood by the listener. Articulatory defects include the misarticulation of both vowels and consonants.

A discussion of the techniques used by the speech therapist in relation to speech conservation is impracticable in the present book. Little research has so far been undertaken into the most appropriate teaching methods relating to speech conservation for adults and the procedures used are mainly those that have been found successful with children. These include the exploitation of residual hearing by suitable amplifying devices such as hearing aids and speech trainers to restore auditory feedback and the use of visual and tactile approaches to monitor and regulate voice quality. A policy statement issued by the British Society of Audiology[11] rightly stresses the importance to adults with a complete or profound hearing loss of kinaesthetic cues for speech conservation. These kinaesthetic cues relate to 'feelings of jaw movement, tongue movement, position of the lips, position of the soft palate, force and control of breath and nasal and laryngeal vibrations'. These kinaesthetic sensations need to be related to such aspects of speech production as the control of voice quality, pitch, intonation, rate and loudness of speech and speech rhythm.

Employment

The handicapping effects of hearing impairment on employment are a major source of anxiety to persons who become deafened or hard of hearing between the ages of school-leaving and retirement. Thomas, Lamont and Harris[12] investigated a sample of 88 adults of employment age with an acquired hearing loss greater than 60 dB. The researchers found that, while the respondents were not likely to be out of work by virtue of their hearing loss, they were experiencing difficulty in coping at work for a variety of reasons categorised under five headings:

1 Dealing with people other than colleagues.
2 Formal work relations.
3 Job proficiency.
4 Social relationships.
5 Loss of status.

It was evident that very many respondents had problems with the telephone and dealing with people other than colleagues (section 1) and that a considerable number had experienced loss of job or job status (section 5).

Difficulties may also be experienced in other areas. Hearing loss may affect job proficiency due to inability to use the telephone or participate in group discussion. Restricted participation in social relationships at work can give rise to feelings of isolation, inadequacy and marginality. There is also the fact that seeking employment becomes more difficult due to the communication problems that arise at interviews and the often negative or unsympathetic attitudes of prospective employers towards the hearing impaired. A person with a hearing impairment experiences a dichotomy of relief at having secured or maintained full-time employment and frustration at the restrictions imposed by the disability on opportunities for advancement or promotion.

Deafened or hard of hearing persons may participate in the services provided by the Employment Service Agency of the Manpower Services Commission that are described in Chapter 8. These include registration on the Disabled Persons Employment Register, assistance from the disablement resettlement officer, assistance towards retraining and, where appropriate, the provision of suitable aids. Disablement resettlement officers do not always understand the differences between the pre-lingually deaf and the deafened and hard of hearing. In dealing with the employment problems of acquired hearing handicap the following aspects should be given special consideration:

1 *What is the client's expectation of working life?* If hearing loss acquires handicapping proportions at the age of 40 the person concerned has some 20–25 years of working life left and some retraining may be advisable. At age 55, however, the emphasis should be on *retaining* employment.

2 *Is the hearing loss progressive?* If this is the case, it is important to estimate the likely effect on employment in say five to ten years time. The client may be able to use the telephone now but will this ability be retained?

3 *How can the existing qualifications, skills and vocational interests of the client be utilised?* Consideration of these factors may indicate opportunities for self-employment, retraining or transferring to other work within the same organisation.

4 *How can the client be assisted to cope with his or her present job?* This may involve strategies developed by or for the client. An exceptional example is that of the adaptation of the Palantype system for use by Jack Ashley in the House of Commons. Most usually this involves the provision of communication aids such as amplified telephones, visual warning systems and similar devices.

5 *Would a change of occupation be desirable due to the psycho-logical strain imposed by hearing impairment?* Where consider-able interaction is involved such as attendance at meetings, discussion and telephone conversations, feelings of strain, inadequacy and loss of confidence may make a change of occupation to less demanding employment beneficial.

For most hearing impaired persons the most prudent course is to stay with their present employer. Employers will often make concessions to existing employees that they would not provide for new workers. Furthermore, both employer and colleagues gradually acquire an understanding of hearing impairment and its consequences so that they can assist the person with a hearing loss. Perhaps this section can best conclude with the observation that there is no simple causal relationship between the severity of hearing loss and its implications for employment. The 'effects' of hearing impairment in the employment of an individual are a complex of clinical, social, psychological and occupational factors.

Family attitudes

The whole family is affected when one member is affected by hearing impairment. The effects listed below are an indicative rather than an exhaustive account of some of the consequences that may arise.

1 The basis of family life is community. Community, in turn, depends on communication. Where one member is unable to participate fully in conversation, for example, at meal-times, he or she may experience feelings of isolation and loneliness. Conversely, hearing members may be conscious of guilt at ignoring the hearing impaired person.

2 Irritability and even hostility may be caused by the frustration of trying to transmit or receive spoken messages. The hearing impaired person may be sensitive to such feelings.

3 As an extension of (2) the hearing impaired person may develop a negative self-image as a burden on the family, due to having to depend on other members for help in oral communication, telephone messages, maintaining friendships and regaining a sense of personal worth.

4 Previously shared interests may be relinquished. A husband and wife, for example, may have enjoyed dancing together or entertaining. When one partner becomes deafened or hard of hearing, he or she may find such activities a strain. A lady known to the writer resented the fact that her husband would not accompany her to church even though he told her repeatedly that the reason was because he could hear so little of the service.

5 Role changes may occur. Severe hearing loss may prevent a housewife from sharing the confidences of her husband and growing children so that difficulties occur in fulfilling the roles of wife and mother. She may, in fact, be relegated to the role of housekeeper.

6 Conflict may arise if requests and instructions are misunderstood. Frequently a hearing impaired person may deny receiving an instruction only to receive the counter-accusation 'You didn't pay attention.'

7   Changes can take place in the personality of the hearing impaired person who appears to become a different individual. Meyerson[13] found that experimentally-induced hearing loss had the following behavioural manifestations: fatigue, irritability, withdrawal from social situations, paranoid reactions such as suspiciousness, inappropriate behaviour, embarrassment and lack of self-confidence.

Because of the above factors it is important that the family of a hearing impaired adult should receive counselling. As Levine[14] has stated:

> The scope of treatment must be broad enough to include not only the patient but also the figures in his life whose attitudes are sufficiently powerful to impede successful adjustment. Immediate family members are figures of major importance. . . . Not infrequently the need for psychotherapy on the part of these persons is greater than the client's.

The same writer points out that where family attitudes are receptive even a hearing impaired person with a less healthy personality has a good chance of coming to terms with his disability. Where, however, family attitudes exhibit rejection, revulsion or misunderstanding even a healthy personality may find it difficult to withstand the effects of serious hearing impairment.

The deafened

Sudden profound hearing impairment is a terrifying and disorientating experience which gives rise to psychological and social consequences, some of which have been mentioned in Chapter 5. It is therefore essential that the person concerned and his or her family should receive immediate constructive assistance and support. Ideally such support should take place in the home area of the person affected. Not all social services departments, however, are able to provide the help needed. There is also the point that: 'To the extent that rehabilitation is also a function of the NHS, the support required by this group (the deafened) does not fall neatly within the existing responsibilities of either health or social services.'[15]

The Link Centre for Deafened People

Registered as a charity in 1972, the Link Centre, in Eastbourne, is the only voluntary body in the UK to arrange courses for adults with a sudden hearing loss. The three aims of the Link Centre are:

1 To give comfort, courage and fresh hope to people who become deafened as adults and to their families.
2 To provide guidelines for their future and to give practical assistance as needed.
3 To draw people together – professionals, deafened people and their families – thus forming a basis for future progress in mutual understanding.

The Link Centre offers a two-week residential course designed to provide an opportunity for the deafened person 'to take stock of the situation, discover new values and goals, perhaps unexpected strengths, talents and unused skills on which to begin to build a new way of living'. As the Director, Rosemary McCall, has wisely said 'The first step in rehabilitation is to survive, to live through the next day.' Only six deafened persons who may be accompanied by members of their family are accepted on any one course. Referral to Link may be by doctors, social workers or by an independent approach to the Centre from the deafened person. The cost of the course at the Link Centre and the travelling involved is usually met by the health authority or social services department sponsoring attendance.

After the course sponsors are provided with a full report and recommendations for the future care of the deafened person. Contact is also maintained with former course members. Without such continuing support much of the benefit of the course will be lost.

The hard of hearing

Surgical rehabilitation and the hearing impairment as it affects the elderly are two aspects of the care of hard of hearing persons that require special consideration.

Surgical rehabilitation

The restoration of hearing to a socially adequate level by surgical means is the most dramatic form of aural rehabilitation. Since World War II the treatment of conductive hearing loss has been revolutionised by the work of otologists who have built on the work of earlier pioneers. Two factors, the development of the operating microscope and the control of infection by antibiotics, have been of particular significance in the success of modern surgery for the relief of conductive hearing loss. Two of the most important of these surgical procedures are *tympanoplasty* and *stapedectomy*.

Tympanoplasty is the term for a group of procedures aimed at eradicating disease and restoring the sound-conducting mechanism of the middle ear. The procedures involved in tympanoplasty may be subdivided into *myringoplasty* and *ossiculoplasty*.

Myringoplasty seeks to repair the ear drum where a perforation is too large to repair by other means. In effect the hole is patched by tissue taken from the temporal muscle. Such repairs can, of course, be made only when the ear is free from discharge.

Ossiculoplasty is the reconstruction of the ossiculor chain, the three small bones of the middle ear popularly termed the hammer, anvil and stapes which may have become immobile or damaged through disease or injury. Destructive disease in the middle ear, for example, most commonly affects the anvil or incus, which, being in the centre of the chain, has the worst blood supply. Here the surgeon may transpose the incus, use a prosthesis to replace part of the chain or even use an ossicle removed from another patient in the course of middle ear surgery.

Stapedectomy, the complete or partial removal of the stapes, is now the standard surgical procedure for the improvement of hearing loss due to otosclerosis. The first stapedectomy involving the use of a prosthesis was performed in 1956 by John Shea Jnr of Tennessee. In his original operation, Shea completely removed the stapes; the oval window was thus left open and its closure was effected by a graft consisting of a small segment of vein removed from the patient's arm. A polythene strut was then used to bridge the gap between the incus and the vein graft. In 1963, Shea began to use a piston made of teflon, a plastic material rather than a polythene strut. Subsequently other types of pistons have been devised, as well as alternatives to vein graft, for closing the oval window.

Stapedectomy does not cure the pathological condition of otosclerosis. It does, however, provide a better than 95 per cent chance of a long-lasting restoration of hearing to a serviceable level in carefully selected cases. The main factor in deciding on the suitability or otherwise of an individual for the operation is the state of the nerve of hearing as shown by the extent to which pure tones are heard better by bone than air conduction. The aim of the operation, in fact, is to close the gap between hearing by bone and air conduction as shown by a pure-tone audiogram. Ideally, the bone-air gap should be between 30 and 60 dB. In about 2 per cent of cases, however, sensorineural loss may occur at the time of the operation or later in 1 per cent of cases after an initially successful result. The otologist will always warn a patient of this risk and that the alternative to a stapedectomy is a hearing aid. There may be little point in encouraging an elderly person who has become well adjusted to a hearing aid to undergo a stapedectomy. It is also because of the slight danger of late sensorineural loss that some otologists believe that it is unwise to operate on both ears. Others believe that at least five years should elapse before an operation on the second ear is contemplated.

Where the improvement obtained from a stapedectomy subsequently deteriorates due to conductive causes, an otologist may possibly perform a revision operation with a reasonable expectation of success. Pearman and Dawes[16] report a conductive failure rate over varying periods of time of approximately 5 per cent of their total stapedectomies, with successful results in 60 per cent of the cases where revision surgery was undertaken.

Hearing impairment and the elderly

The incidence of hearing impairment mainly due to presby-acusis rises steeply in the older age groups. An estimate is that about one-in-three persons over 65 has a significant hearing loss and two-in-three of those aged 80 and above.

Elderly hearing impaired persons are, of course, found both in the community and in residential accommodation for the elderly.

The results derived by Herbst and Humphrey[17] from a study aimed at ascertaining whether the high incidence of hearing impairment thought to exist in the elderly population is related to the high prevalence of mental disorder known to be found in the post-70 age group are important since, for the first time, audiometry was used by the researchers to measure the incidence of 'deafness' among old people living in the community. 'Deafness' was defined as 'an average loss over speech frequencies (at 1 kHz, 2 kHz and 4 kHz) of 35 dB or more in the better ear'. The prevalence of hearing loss at various ages of a sample of 253 out of 365 persons aged 70 and over, living at home and registered with the central surgery of an Inner London group practice, is shown in Chapter 1, p.8. Other findings from this survey are listed below:

1   There is a significant relationship between hearing impairment in the elderly and social class: the incidence of hearing loss being higher in the lower socio-economic groups.

2   Unlike some other studies on presbyacusis which have shown better hearing in women than men, Herbst and Humphrey found no significant differences between the proportions of men and women who were hearing impaired.

3   Many respondents did not report hearing difficulties to their general practitioner although they paid frequent visits about other chronic disorders. This apathy suggests that both patients and doctors may passively accept hearing loss as a normal part of ageing for which little can be done.

4   Some general practitioners may not refer patients for a hearing aid because they are pessimistic about the benefits to be obtained by elderly patients. The majority of respondents in the sample, however, found a hearing aid helpful.

5   Doctors and other health professionals might be more alert to the existence of hearing loss in elderly patients if they were more aware of the incidence of the disability in these age groups. The problem lies in recognising the existence of hearing problems where these are not mentioned by the patient.

Apart from general physical, psychological, social and economic considerations, the ability of an elderly impaired person to live in the community will be influenced by such factors as:

1   The understanding and support received from family, neighbours and social workers for the deaf.

2   The capacity to cope with the isolation and loneliness consequent on hearing loss.

3   The availability and use made of such rehabilitative measures as speech-reading, auditory training and hearing and environmental aids.

Studies by Martin and Peckford[18] and Burton[19], both using audiometry, have been made of hearing impaired residents in homes for the elderly.

Martin and Peckford's sample comprised 425 persons aged from under 65 (5.4%) to 90+ (12.9%). The numbers with a hearing loss in the better ear, less than 30 dB, 30–59 dB and 60+ dB were 83 (19.5%), 257 (60.5%) and 85 (20%) respectively. Of those with a loss of 60+ dB, 32 (37.6%) and 43 (50.6%) were in the 75–84 and 86+ age groups. This study is significant for three reasons.

Firstly it highlights the danger that hearing impaired residents may be overlooked. Staff in charge of homes or their senior colleagues were asked to identify persons who had difficulty hearing and understanding most things people say without seeing their face or lips. After subsequent audiometry it was found that 27.1 per cent of the severely hearing impaired (i.e. with a loss of 60+ dB) had not been recognised as such. Hearing aid owners (not necessarily users), women and those admitting to their handicap were more likely to be identified than their counterparts. Persons longest in residence were, not surprisingly, more likely to be identified as having a hearing loss than those who had been in the homes for a shorter period.

Secondly, the study provides useful information regarding the needs of hearing impaired elderly residents. More than a quarter of the sample had wax in one or both ears. Some elderly persons needed to be assessed for a hearing aid. Half the instruments already fitted were either not working or required specialist attention; in other cases instruction was required in the use and maintenance of the aid.

A general need was identified for homes to be fitted with a television loop system. Some residents would have benefited from personal television adaptors and the availability of RNID television play synopses. Speech-reading instruction, speech therapy and social interaction such as visits by volunteers or the opportunity of joining a nearby hard of hearing club were other ways in which hearing impaired persons could be helped. For many residents, however, the most significant need was that staff should either be skilful in communicating with the hearing impaired or use a device such as the communicator described in Chapter 10.

Thirdly, the researchers emphasise the importance of specialist training not only for the staff of homes, but also for others such as social workers involved in assessment and admission. Such training might have the following aims:

1   To stimulate interest in hearing impairment and hearing impaired persons.

2 To provide a better understanding of the physical and psychological implications of hearing impairment.

3 To enable staff to recognise quickly hearing impaired persons and the circumstances in which specialised help should be sought.

4 To show staff what non-specialist help they can give or organise with special emphasis on skill in communicating with hearing impaired people.

In this connection a training package[20] produced by the DHSS in 1977 is very useful. Other training programmes are suggested in a publication of Age Concern[21].

Burton[19] investigated a sample of 148 hearing impaired residents in five local authority homes for the elderly supplemented by a questionnaire to the wardens of a further 60 hostels. The questionnaire used and responses obtained are of interest to all concerned with the welfare of elderly persons in residential accommodation (Table 9.6).

Finally, the habilitation of elderly persons with an acquired hearing loss is significantly influenced by the attitudes of both clients and those responsible for their welfare. A negative attitude on the part of the client to procedures designed to assist in overcoming hearing impairment may be due to an inability to accept the changes of old age or to view the future positively, e.g. 'Why should I bother about a hearing aid at my age?' Negative attitudes may also be displayed by participants in the habilitation process. Remarks by a general practitioner such as 'What can you expect at your age?' are not constructive. Others concerned with habilitation may find it difficult to act positively to cases where little or no progress is being made and the client is unco-operative. Rudd and Margolin[22] have stressed the importance of maintenance therapy with geriatric clients. The aim of maintenance therapy is to utilise procedures which may retard the degeneration of chronically ill patients by attempting either to arrest or to slow down the process even though this may only be temporary. Hearing and environmental aids, speech-reading and auditory training, joining in the activities of hard of hearing clubs, regular visitation and a patient and constructive attitude on the part of all concerned with the services provided for hearing impaired persons may all be applications of maintenance therapy.

Table 9.6 Questionnaire for wardens in local authority homes

Question	Response
1 Is deafness entered on the residents' record cards?	Yes – 43%
2 Have any of the staff had instruction on overcoming the problems of deafness?	Yes – 48%
3 Does the hostel have any tactile fire alarms?	No response given to this question
4 Do you (i.e. the hostel) have a stock of leaflets on clear speech for lip-reading?	Yes – 11%
5 Is there a stock in the hostel of batteries, cords and purses for hearing aids?	Batteries – 43% Cords – 35% Purses – 5%
6 Does the hostel have (a) a television listening aid? (b) a radio listening aid? (c) personal communication aid?	Television aid – 6% Radio aid – 3% Communicator – Yes 37%
7 Is the general practitioner invited to examine the ears of residents for the presence of wax?	Yes – 79%
8 Do staff ensure that the ear mould of residents' hearing aids are washed and cleaned?	Yes – 65%
9 Does the hotel get copies of television play synopses?	Yes – 9%
10 Does the specialist social worker for the deaf from the local voluntary service for the deaf or social services department (a) Visit the hostel to advise the warden? (b) Provide a regular visiting service for any of the residents?	Visit by social worker – 6% Regular visitation to residents – 2%

References

1 Levine, Edna Simon. *The Psychology of Deafness*, Columbia University Press, New York, 1960, pp. 259–265.

2 Davis, H. 'The Articulation Area and the Social Adequacy Index for Hearing', *Laryngoscope*, Vol. 58, 1948, pp. 761–778.

3 Alpiner, J. (Ed.). *Handbook of Adult Rehabilitative Audiology*, Williams and Wilkins Co., Baltimore, 1978.

4 High, W., Fairbanks, G. and Glorig. 'Scale for self-assessment of hearing handicap,' *Journal of Speech and Hearing Disorders*, Vol. 29, 1964, pp. 215–230.

5 Ewertsen, H. and Birk-Nielsen, H. 'Social Hearing Handicap Index', *Audiology*, Vol. 12, 1973, pp. 180–187.

6 Noble, W. and Atherley, G. 'The Hearing Measurement Scale: A questionnaire for the assessment of auditory disability, *Journal of Audiological Research*, Vol. 10, 1970, pp. 229–250.

7 Barcham and Stephens. 'The Use of an open-ended problems Questionnaire in Auditory Rehabilitation', *British Journal of Audiology*, Vol. 14, 1980, pp. 49–54.

8 Wood, S. 'Maskers and Tinnitus Patients,' *British Tinnitus Association Newsletter* No. 17, July 1982.

9 Irlam, Wechsler and Parker. 'Speech Therapy for Hearing Impaired Adults in Great Britain', *Hearing Aid Journal* (USA).

10 Brown, B. B. *Speech Therapy – Principles and Practice.* Churchill Livingstone, 1981, Ch. 11, p. 212.

11 Markides, Brooks, Hart and Stephens. 'The Rehabilitation of Hearing Impaired Adults (Policy of the British Society of Audiology)', *British Journal of Audiology*, No. 13, 1979, p. 11.

12 Thomas, Lamont and Harris. 'Problems Encountered at Work by People with Severe Acquired Hearing Loss', *British Journal of Audiology*, Vol. 16, 1982, pp. 39–43.

13 Meyerson, L. 'Experimental Injury: An Approach to the Dynamics of Disability', *Journal of Social Issues*, Vol. 4, 1948, pp. 68–71.

14 Levine, Edna A. *The Psychology of Deafness*, Columbia University Press, 1960, Ch. 4, pp. 90–91.

15 DHSS. *Report of a Sub-Committee Appointed to Consider the Role of Social Services in the Care of the Deaf of All Ages*, June 1977.

16 Pearman, K. and Dawes, J. D. K. 'Post-stapedectomy Conductive Deafness and the Results of Revision Surgery', *Journal of Laryngology and Otology*, Vol. 96, May 1982, pp. 405–410.

17 Herbst, K. G. and Humphrey, C. 'Prevalence of Hearing Impairment in the Elderly Living at Home', *Journal of the Royal College of General Practitioners*, March 1981, pp. 155–158.

18 Martin, D. and Peckford, B. 'Hearing Impairment in Homes for the Elderly' *Social Work Service*, Vol. 17, 1978, pp. 52–62.

19 Burton, D. K. 'Hearing Impaired Residents in Local Authority Homes for the Elderly', Address to the North Regional Association for the Deaf, 14 April 1977. Typewritten.

20 DHSS. *Staff Development Package on Acquired Deafness*, 1977, HMSO.

21 Nattrass, Susan. *Sound Sense. How local groups can help hard of hearing people*, Age Concern, 1982.

22 Rudd and Margolin. *Maintenance Therapy for the Geriatric Patient.* C. C. Thomas, 1968.

Chapter 10

Hearing and environmental aids

Amplification of speech by means of a suitable hearing aid is for the majority of hearing impaired persons the most important element in their habilitation or rehabilitation. This chapter explains the main components of a hearing aid, the types of aid available and some important factors relating to their procurement, prescription and use. A description of some other environmental aids is also given.

Hearing aids

What is a hearing aid?

A hearing aid is an amplifying device specifically designed for assisting hearing impaired persons to achieve better receptive communication. It has been stated that the oldest, cheapest and most readily accessible aid to hearing is the cupped hand behind the ear. In this way, the sound level at the ear can be raised by about 6 dB. Goldstein[1] in a historical survey has categorised devices designed to improve hearing into six groups: hearing tubes; ear-trumpets; concealed or camouflaged sound receptors, e.g. acoustic chairs, fans, hats etc; devices to increase the size and capacity of parts of the sound-conducting mechanism, e.g. artificial external ears (auricles) and artificial ear-drums; non-electric bone-conduction devices, e.g. strips of wood, metal or vulcanite to conduct sound through the skull; electronic aids.

Some of the above have been practically valueless. Others, especially hearing tubes and ear-trumpets, known as acoustic aids, are especially useful with elderly deaf persons who have difficulty with electronic aids and are available, when prescribed by an otologist, from an NHS hearing aid clinic.

Electronic hearing aids

It is, however, an electronic hearing aid that most people think about when considering how they can compensate for a hearing loss. As shown in Fig. 10.1, a hearing aid has four main components: a microphone, an amplifier, an earphone and the power supply. The ear-mould, while not strictly part of the aid, is also an important element in its efficiency.

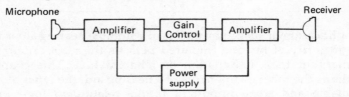

Fig. 10.1 The main components of a hearing aid

The microphone

The microphone changes or transduces the energy carried by sound waves into electrical energy. This is done by means of a diaphragm which is made to vibrate by the sound waves very much like the ear-drum in the human ear.

The amplifier

The function of the amplifier located inside the aid is to increase the rather weak electrical signal produced by the microphone. The magnitude of this increase is determined by the gain control setting and limited by the maximum power output of the instrument (see p. 127 for a definition of gain). Amplification is effected in several stages. Generally, the more stages of amplification the greater the intensity or sound energy of the signal reaching the receiver.

The receiver

The role of the receiver is to convert back into acoustic wave form the electrical signal magnified many times by the amplifier. It therefore reverses the function of the microphone. Most receivers are air-conductive and may be external or internal. An external receiver of the so-called 'button' type used with body-worn aids is connected directly to the ear-mould. The internal receiver used with behind-the-ear aids is located with the amplifier inside the case of the instrument, the amplified signal being conveyed to the ear-mould by a tube.

Where there is an ear discharge, or a very significant bone-air gap a bone-conduction receiver may be fitted. A bone-conduction earphone is essentially a vibrator which is placed against the mastoid so that sound can be transmitted into the inner ear. The disadvantage of bone-conduction earphones which are used only with body-worn and spectacle aids is that they require more power with a subsequent increase in battery consumption, they transmit a narrow range of frequencies and, in body aids, a headband must be worn to ensure an adequate pressure on the mastoid.

The power supply

The battery or cell (strictly the term battery applies to two or more cells) is the heart of the hearing aid since it provides the power. Hearing aid batteries fall into three broad categories:

Carbon-zinc or Leclanché batteries similar to those used in pen torches, are used for body aids. These have the advantage of low cost but are not rechargeable. Their output gradually diminishes and the user has therefore some warning before the battery is completely spent.

Mercury or 'button'-type batteries are used for behind-the-ear aids. Although the initial cost is higher than for their carbon-zinc counterparts, mercury batteries last longer and, for this reason, ultimately work out cheaper. Mercury batteries maintain a uniform voltage until almost exhausted. Some users find the absence of warning before the cut-out a disadvantage. If not completely run down, these batteries can be recharged.

The third type of battery, the genuinely *rechargeable cell,* is made of combinations of metal such as nickel and cadmium or silver and zinc. Such cells do not generate electricity but absorb current from a battery charger in a similar way to a car battery accumulating current from the dynamo. These cells can be recharged up to 100 times and will last for about 12 months. Even though it is necessary to buy four batteries initially – one for the aid, one to keep in reserve and two to keep on charge – they are the most economical way of powering a hearing aid over a year.

Details of suppliers of battery chargers can be obtained from the Scientific and Technical Department of the RNID.

The ear-mould

The primary function of the ear-mould is to direct sound to the ear passage. The ear-mould also supports the air-conduction receiver of a body aid or fixes an ear-level aid securely to the head of the wearer. The performance and comfort of a hearing aid is significantly affected by the ear-mould and for this reason the design, manufacture and modification of this component is a minor specialism. If an airtight fit is not secured, some of the amplification will be lost before it reaches the ear-drum and there will be embarassing whistling from acoustic feedback.

An ill-fitting mould may also cause chafing of the ear passage making the aid uncomfortable to wear. With a 'button'-type receiver acoustic feedback can sometimes be remedied by placing a piece of 'Blu-tack' between the face of the receiver and the face of the ear-mould ensuring, of course, that the sound tube is unblocked.

Young children may, due to the growth of their ears, require a new ear-mould several times a year. As they become older, the intervals for the replacement of the ear-mould become longer.

Auditory trainers and individual hearing aids

Auditory trainers and individual hearing aids operate on the same electronic principles but they differ in that the latter, as the name implies, are training devices used mainly in group situations rather than for personal everyday use. Figure 10.2 shows the main amplification devices, other than environmental aids, used in the rehabilitation of hearing impaired persons.

Auditory trainers

Two important factors influencing the successful use of any amplifying device are the distance of the sound source from the receiver and the acoustic conditions obtaining in a given situation. As has already been stated, sound fades as it travels through the air, its intensity diminishing as the square of the distance from its source. In simple terms, this means that if a speaker 2ft away moves to a distance of 4ft, his voice will sound

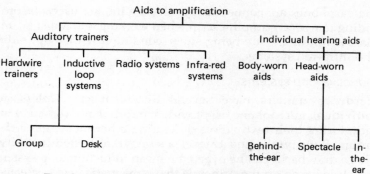

Fig. 10.2 The main non-environmental amplification devices

not half but only one quarter as loud as it did before. Acoustic conditions usually referred to as the 'signal-to-noise ratio' (S/N) ratio, relates to the difference between the decibel level of the source signal, in this case, speech, and the background noise in which it occurs. If the source signal is greater in intensity than the background noise by, say 10 dB, we have a positive S/N ratio of 10 dB. The higher the positive number or the quieter the environment, the more favourable the conditions for hearing. In group conditions, such as a class-room, other acoustic conditions detrimental to a hearing aid user, such as reverberation from the wall surfaces, will also apply. In such group conditions, simply increasing amplification will not only magnify the voice of the speaker but also background noise. A reduction of a negative S/N ratio can be obtained if the hearing aid microphone can be placed as closely as possible to the person speaking. It is the application of this principle that auditory trainers used in group situations are designed to achieve.

Hardwire trainers

With group trainers the teacher speaks into a microphone wired to a large amplifier that delivers the amplified speech to several sets of earphones. These earphones, usually in headsets, are wired to the amplifier and the speech reception level can be adjusted by an individual control box located on the pupil's desk by which the gain and tone delivered to each ear can be regulated.

Desk trainers, which are portable, with the microphone, amplifier and battery all contained in the carrying case to which the earphones are connected by a hard wire, are useful in providing temporary amplification when working with one person. Hardwire trainers are being superseded rapidly by loop, radio and infra-red systems.

Inductive loop systems

Hardwire trainers have several disadvantages. Unless an individual microphone is provided pupils have difficulty in monitoring their own voices or hearing other members of the group. Both pupils and teacher also have restricted mobility. These drawbacks can be overcome by an induction loop system which is based on the principle that a magnetic field is created around a wire proportional to the electric current flowing through the wire. To produce the magnetic field more easily, the wire carrying the amplified signal from the teacher's microphone is looped around the room.

The pupil wears a personal hearing aid fitted with an induction coil which induces an equivalent pattern of current in the aid. This electro-magnetic input is then amplified and fed to the receiver of the aid where it is transduced into sound waves for delivery to the ear.

Induction loop systems have the advantages of pupil-teacher mobility and by the use of their own aids, enable pupils to select the most suitable level of amplification. The main disadvantages relate to variations in the electro-magnetic signal within a looped room and 'overspill'. This latter term refers to the fact that the magnetic field extends beyond the loop so that hearing aid users in adjacent rooms will pick up the signals if they are switched to the loop position.

Induction loops are not confined to class-room use but can be utilised in churches or theatres or within the home to enable a hearing impaired person to listen to radio or television.

Frequency modulated (FM) radio frequency training units

These systems, such as the Phonic Ear, have far greater flexibility than either of those described above. Operating on batteries and receiving radio signals from the atmosphere they require no loop or wires and can therefore be used in any room or out of doors. Because there is no installation of any kind, such a system can be used to integrate a hearing impaired pupil into a class of hearing children or used by the child at home. In effect the teacher's microphone is a miniature radio transmitter broadcasting on any of the 12 frequencies or channels specified by the Home Office. The pupil's receiver, tuned to the same frequency as the teacher's microphone, may either be a special radio microphone hearing aid or a small radio receiver that connects to the user's personal hearing aid.

Infra-red systems

These use a beam of infra-red light to transmit the teacher's voice rather than radio signals. This obviates overspill and enables all aids to operate on one frequency. The main disadvantage is that such aids cannot be used out of doors since sunlight contains infra-red which causes interference with reception.

Individual hearing aids

Individual hearing aids, described below, are usually categorised according to whether they are worn on the body or the head. Three types of head-worn aids: behind-the-ear, spectacle and in-the-ear may be identified. Cochlear implants, prosthetic devices designed to replace the cochlear hair cells in cases of profound sensory hearing impairment are still at an experimental stage and are not referred to in this book.

Body-worn aids

Because of their larger size which enabled larger batteries to be used and the incorporation of more sophisticated controls, body-worn aids were always prescribed for severely hearing impaired persons for whom a high-powered aid was essential. This is no longer necessary but there are still certain classes of users for whom a body-worn aid with its larger controls and robust construction is particularly suitable. These include very young children, elderly persons with impaired vision or poor eye-hand co-ordination, and those with poor manual dexterity due to rheumatism or similar causes. Two other advantages of this type of aid are that it can be attached securely to the user's clothing and that because the microphone and receiver are two components separated from each other by 10–20 in., acoustic feedback is minimised.

The main disadvantages relate to clothes rub and the difficulty of achieving binaural amplification.

Clothes rub, caused by the microphone rubbing against the clothes of the wearer, can be distracting. In some aids this is minimised by placing the microphone on top of the case. It can also be reduced by the use of a suede plastic pocket with a rustle-free lining. Such a pocket is obtainable at small cost from the RNID.

Behind-the-ear aids

These are now the most popular type of aid. All the components of the instrument are contained in a plastic case worn behind the ear. Amplified sound is conveyed from the receiver to the ear-mould by a translucent tube. The microphone may face either forwards or rearwards. For most hearing situations the forward-facing microphone is preferable since it tends to eliminate partially unwanted sound generated behind the head. Because of their small size, behind-the-ear aids are very inconspicuous and, with women, can be completed concealed by an appro-priate hair-style. Clothes rub is also eliminated. The principal disadvantage is that acoustic feedback may occur even at relatively low gain levels due to the close proximity of the microphone and receiver.

Spectacle aids

With this type of aid the microphone, amplifier and receiver are built into either one or both arms of the spectacle frame. Binaural hearing can be provided if an aid is in both arms. This arrange-ment is preferable to two body-worn aids as it allows natural head movements. The frames are also ideal for use in connection with 'bi-unilateral' hearing aids. These, known by the acronyms CROS and BICROS, are designed to assist people with a hearing loss in one ear or those with little or no residual hearing in one ear and a less severe loss in the other. The primary goal is to improve the hearing of speech originating on the side of the weaker ear. The effect is to give the user a form of binaural hearing even when one ear is non-functional so that the direction from which a sound is coming is more readily detectable.

CROS stands for contralateral routing of signals. In this arrangement the microphone and amplifier are on one side of the head with wiring leading to the receiver on the other side. As shown earlier, the closer the proximity of the microphone to the receiver, the greater the likelihood of acoustic feedback. With the CROS arrangement not only are the two components separated but the head also acts as a buffer so that feedback is reduced.

BICROS (bilateral contralateral routing of signals) is for people who have a bilateral loss with usable residual hearing in only one ear. In this arrangement two microphones are used, one on each side of the head, with a receiver in one ear. The sounds picked up by each microphone are fed into a mixer unit that combines them before they are amplified and transmitted to the usable ear. While both CROS and BICROS arrangements are not confined to spectacle aids and can be used with both behind-the-ear and in-the-ear aids, the spectacle aid has obvious advantages.

Apart from the high cost and the fact that removal of the glasses means removal of the aid, spectacle aids have the disadvantage that maintenance problems are higher than with any other type of aid. Even a simple adjustment to ensure better fitting of the spectacles can be difficult when the frames contain electronic circuitry.

All-in-the-ear aids

Often described in advertisements as 'clarifiers' or 'correctors' these are the smallest type of aid available, all the components being connected to or integrated with the ear-mould. Formerly these aids were only suitable for a mild hearing loss and the fact that the microphone and receiver were close together resulted in considerable acoustic feedback. These disadvantages have now been largely overcome and a high gain can be provided but they are still not adequate for a user with a severe hearing loss. The location of the microphone on the outside of the ear facing in the same direction as the auditory canal takes advantage of the sound-focusing function of the auricle. All in-the-ear aids are not invisible and may be more conspicuous than behind-the-ear aids. The controls may also pose difficulties for elderly or physically handicapped wearers.

Obtaining a hearing aid

Hearing aids may be obtained on free loan from a hearing aid clinic under the National Health Service or bought privately from a hearing aid dispenser.

Government provided aids

At the time of writing (1982) the original OL series of mainly body-worn aids is virtually obsolete and in process of being replaced by the behind-the-ear BE10 range. The instruments numbers BE/11/12/13/14 and 15 are probably capable of satisfying about 70 per cent of the hearing impaired population. A fairly high-powered, body-worn aid, the BW61, is also available. Acoustic aids such as speaking tubes and ear-trumpets can also be issued under NHS provision.

An adult wishing to obtain an NHS aid must ask his general practitioner to refer him to an otologist at a hospital ENT Department. If the otologist considers that the patient will benefit from the use of a hearing aid an instrument will be issued by the hearing aid clinic.

For children, responsibility for the prescription of a hearing aid also rests with the consultant otologist who may seek the advice of an audiologist. Up to the age of 18 (21 if continuing in full-time education) the range of standard NHS aids is supplemented by some six commercial aids (three body-worn and three post-aural) available under 'call off' arrangements made with the suppliers by the DHSS. If, in the opinion of the otologist, there is no suitable instrument either within the NHS or 'call off' contract range, the health authority at its discretion, may purchase any commercially available aid. It is also possible for the otologist to prescribe two aids if he considers this to be desirable.

Batteries and repairs in respect of NHS aids are free for both adults and children. The same applies to commercial aids bought by health authorities for children and young people until the users reach the upper age limits of 18 or 21. A useful booklet on NHS hearing aids is obtainable from the RNID.

Commercial aids

In addition to a government aid there is nothing to prevent an individual from buying a commercial aid from a hearing aid dispenser. There are three advantages of owning both a government and a commercial aid.

Firstly, a spare aid ensures that the user is not inconvenienced should the NHS aid be out-of-commission for repairs. While the NHS clinic is usually able to supply a replacement aid from stock, it is only authorised to issue spare aids to deaf-blind persons.

Secondly, government aids are designed to meet the needs of the majority of users and the range of choice is therefore small in contrast with the wide range of commercial aids. It may be possible for a dispenser to fit an aid more suited to the requirements of an individual user. Thirdly, NHS electronic aids are confined to the body-worn and behind-the-ears types. All-in-the-ear and spectacle models are only available as commercial aids.

Commercial aids, however, are not cheap either from the standpoints of capital outlay or the running costs of batteries, repairs and depreciation. A commercial aid may, according to its usage, have a useful life of 5–7 years. The following advice to prospective purchasers of commercial aids taken from the author's earlier book *Your Hearing Loss and How to Cope With It*, may usefully be repeated:

Before trying to find a (hearing aid) dealer you would be wise to do two things. Firstly, if you have not already done so, ask your doctor to refer you to an otologist. This advice is worth reiterating since it may be that appropriate treatment would remove the need for an aid. Secondly, if you *do* need an aid, start by writing to the RNID and asking for their list of hearing aids. This publication will provide you with particulars of the names, descriptions and prices of the majority of hearing aids on the market. . . .

Apart from this general advice some of the following hints may also be useful.

Try to locate a dealer within reasonable distance of your home to save unnecessary expense and inconvenience should your aid require after-sales service.

Don't buy from a travelling exhibition unless the supplier can provide acceptable after-sales facilities in your area.

Tell the dispenser the type of aid you would prefer e.g. behind-the-ear, spectacle, etc. and how much you want to pay. Let him know where the aid will usually be worn, e.g. in the home, in a noisy factory etc.

A good dispenser will test your ability to discriminate speech sounds as well as pure tones. A *WHICH* survey in 1973 reported that less than half of their respondents had been tested by speech audiometry.

Do not expect a hearing aid dispenser to prescribe with the same precision as an optician. He will generally categorise your loss as 'mild', 'moderate', or 'severe' and select aids from his stock which he believes to be appropriate.

Make allowances for some distortion and oscillation when you try an aid with a *standard* ear mould. An *individual* ear mould will almost certainly improve reception.

Before purchasing ask the dispenser whether you may try the aid for a few days at home, either free or on the basis of a returnable deposit. If a trial on such terms is refused you are well advised not to buy.

While the aid is in your possession, treat it carefully, test it fairly and, if you decide not to purchase, return it promptly either in person or by registered post.

Only *you* can decide which aid is more satisfactory from the standpoints of comfort, speech intelligibility and tone quality. Do not be masterminded into buying any other aid.

Do not pay more than you need for an aid. Ask about a discount, particularly if you are paying cash. If you have previously used a hearing aid, ascertain whether the dispenser will give a 'trade in' for your old instrument. The allowance may be small, but a useful contribution to the cost of your new aid.

When buying an aid it is reasonable to expect one year's guarantee covering repairs.

For many years the hearing aid industry had a poor public image due to the activities of high-pressure salesmen who had few scruples about exploiting prospective clients who were desperate for help with their impaired hearing. When introducing the Hearing Aid Council Bill in 1968, Laurie Pavitt declared that his purpose was 'to protect the hard of hearing from the hard selling' and to 'put service, education and information in the place of gimmick sales promotion'. The enactment of the Hearing Aid Council Act 1968 and the rules laid down by the *Advertising Standards Authority* relating to hearing aid advertisements and exhibitions have done much to provide better protection for the purchasers of hearing aids.

The main responsibilities of the *Hearing Aid Council* established in 1969 by the Board of Trade are:

1 To provide for the registration within the Council of all dispensers selling hearing aids and all employers of such dispensers. It is now illegal for unregistered individuals, partnerships or companies to sell hearing aids. The Disciplinary Committee of the Council has power to remove the name of any registered person or body corporate from the register.

2 To lay down standards of competence for hearing aid dispensers and those wishing to take up the occupation.

3 To lay down a Code of Trade Practice for adoption by registered dispensers and employees of dispensers. (This Code is reproduced in Appendix 1.)

The *Advertising Standards Authority,* established in 1962, is independent of the advertising industry although it is financed by the Advertising Association. The Authority adjudicates on general advertising issues, deals with complaints from the public and investigates action or non-action on reported breaches of the British Code of Advertising Practice. The Code lays down the following rules for advertisements relating to hearing aids and hearing aid exhibitions:

8.17   *Hearing Aids*

    8.17.1   Where an advertisement states the prices of a hearing aid the advertiser should specify the upper and lower limits of his overall price range.

    8.17.2   The names of hearing aids should not in themselves exaggerate the product's effectiveness (e.g. such names as 'Magic Sound' and 'Miracle Ear' are not acceptable.

    8.17.3   Advertisements for hearing aids on a rental basis are subject to rules applying to hire of domestic appliances.

8.18   *Hearing Aid Exhibitions*

    8.18.1   Advertisements for such exhibitions should only be accepted where the organiser has given an undertaking that:

      a   he will ensure the presence of at least one registered dispenser at all times throughout the period the exhibition is open;

      b   he will offer for inspection a comprehensive range of models of hearing aids;

      c   he will make available for purposes of testing at least one pure tone *and* one speech audiometer.

    8.18.2   The full name and address of the advertiser's head office should be prominently stated in any advertisement for a hearing aid show or exhibition, and no impression should be given that such events are other than commercially promoted.

Personnel concerned with the selection of a hearing aid

Within the National Health Service the fitting of hearing aids and ear-moulds forms a substantial part of the duties of a physiological measurement technician (audiology) who may undertake additional responsibilities such as diagnostic audiometry, vestibular function tests, teaching and adminis-tration. NHS aids can only be obtained if the client has seen an otologist who, subject to his (the consultant's) approval, leaves such decisions as the selection of the model, the choice of ear and the fitting of an ear-mould to the PMT(A). In 1979 a sub-committee appointed to review the training and qualifications of PMTS(A) recommended that entry to the grade of technician would be conditional upon a student obtaining an Ordinary National Certificate in Science of the Technician Education Council and also successfully completing a professional examination organised by the Audiology Technician's Group (ATG) of the *British Society of Audiology*. Concurrently with study for these qualifications the student is required to receive in-service training at a centre approved by the ATG.

In the private sector, applicants for registration as dispensers under the Hearing Aid Council Act are required to pass written and practical examinations set by the Council. Qualifying examinations for membership are also held by the *Society of Hearing Aid Audiologists*. *The Guild of Hearing Aid Specialists* is an association of hearing aid dispensers who are prepared to adhere to a code imposing higher professional standards on its members than those prescribed by the Hearing Aid Council. *The Hearing Aid Industry Association* is the trade association for all sections of the private hearing aid industry.

Selection of a Hearing Aid

Selection by a PMT(A) or hearing aid dispenser of the most suitable aid or aids for a particular client should be preceded by an examination by an otologist. In the NHS this will be routine. In the private sector the Code of Practice issued by the Hearing Aid Council requires non-medically qualified dispensers to advise a client to seek medical advice if this has not already been done where there has been exposure to loud noise or any of the following conditions: excessive wax, aural discharge, vertigo, earache, deafness of short duration or sudden onset, unilateral perceptive deafness, conductive hearing loss, tinnitus.

Indications as to the prognosis for successful hearing aid use and the most appropriate instrument are also provided by pure-tone and speech audiometry. Berger and Millin[2] state that an audiogram showing a flat, gradually rising or gradually falling, pure-tone threshold contour represents the most favourable prediction of success while the converse will result where a sharp drop occurs at any of the lower frequencies. Similarly word discrimination scores under headphones provide a good prediction of the likely success with an aid and the choice of ear for fitment. An unaided score of 90 per cent or higher suggests that amplification will give good results while scores lower than 50 per cent indicate a probability of only limited success with amplification.

Three important considerations in the selection of an aid are the type and severity of the hearing impairment, and personal factors relating to the potential user.

Type and severity of hearing impairment

A hearing aid is most easily fitted in case of pure conductive impairment where the principal consideration is gain. Gain may be defined as the output of the aid at the receiver minus the input at the microphone. If at 1,000 Hz the output of the aid is 100 dB and the input 60 dB then, at the stated frequency the gain is 40 dB. The amount of gain delivered is regulated by the volume control which can usually be moved to any of up to ten positions. Hearing aids may be categorised as providing 'mild' (25–40 dB), 'moderate' (40–55 dB) or 'high' (60 dB+) gain.

With sensorineural or mixed impairment, recruitment, which is not associated with conductive loss, may complicate the selection of an instrument. Recruitment is an exaggerated sensation of hearing following a slight increase in the intensity of sound. Where recruitment is present the margin between the SRT (speech reception threshold) and overloading the cochlea may be small. Three controls developed to minimise the effects of recruitment are AVC (Automatic Volume Control), PC (Peak Clipping) and DRC (Dynamic Range Compression).

The function of the *Automatic Volume Control* is to limit the maximum output of the amplifier so that irrespective of the input level, the output can never exceed a predetermined volume which is below the user's threshold of pain.

Peak Clipping cuts off peak intensities whenever they exceed a pre-set output limit.

Dynamic Range Compression like AVC and PC is intended to control sound pressures to a level below that at which discomfort and distortion is experienced. Unlike AVC and PC, which are limited to a fixed-output sound pressure, DRC is linked to a fixed-input sound pressure level.

Personal factors relating to the user

These include physical conditions such as arthritis which may make it difficult for a client to insert batteries or operate the controls of an instrument, the motivation of the prospective user and the conditions in which the aid will normally be worn.

Deciding which ear to fit

The success of an aid may be diminished by fitting it in the wrong ear. The choice of ear will be determined on the basis of information obtained from pure-tone and speech discrimination testing but some broad guidelines are as follows:

1 Fit the ear with the best speech discrimination score and the largest dynamic range.
2 Fit the poorer ear where the average pure-tone loss at 1,000, 1,500 and 2,000 Hz in the better ear is not worse than 40 dB and the average at the same frequencies in the poorer ear is not greater than 60 dB. This arrangement enables the unaided better ear to contribute to the total auditory signal received by the client.
3 Where both ears are approximately the same in terms of speech discrimination and dynamic range, select the ear with the flattest, pure-tone threshold contour as shown by the audiogram.
4 If the client can use the telephone without the assistance of an aid, fit the right ear for right-handed persons and the converse for those who are left-handed. This arrangement gives the free use of the dominant hand for writing etc.

Binaural fitting

Binaural fitting means the use of two distinct hearing aids. The use of two receivers attached by a Y-shaped cord to a single amplifier provides bilateral stimulation rather than binaural hearing. Since World War II the use of two aids has been advocated to exploit the residual hearing of children. On the basis that two normal ears are better than one, a growing number of adults are choosing to use two aids of the in-the-ear or behind-the-ear types. In Denmark between 60 per cent and 70 per cent of adult hearing aid users have an aid in each ear. Advantages claimed for the use of two aids include improved speech discrimination in noisy surroundings, better location of sound direction and an enhanced subjective appreciation of auditory space. Markides[3] states that the most suitable candidates for binaural aid fittings are people 'with fairly symmetrical bilateral hearing impairment ranging from 50 dB to 100 dB with the following exceptions:

1   People with a relatively flat impairment in one ear and with a steep high frequency loss in the other ear;
2   People suffering from diplacusis (the hearing of the same sound differently by one ear from the way it is heard by the other);
3   Elderly people with severe fine manipulation problems.

Using a hearing aid

A booklet entitled *General Guidance to Hearing Aid Users* is issued with every NHS aid. Some similar publication is also given to purchasers of commercial aids. It needs to be stressed, however, that a period of adjustment will be necessary before the maximum benefit will be obtained from the instrument. As McCall[4] rightly observes, 'Spectacles take a few days, false teeth a few weeks but hearing aids may take many, many months.' There is evidence that many people who have been issued with a hearing aid do not, without encouragement, persevere in its use. A study by Brooks[5] of persons supplied with body-worn aids at NHS hearing aid clinics on an 'over-the-counter' basis demonstrated that within a year around 30 per cent had given up using the aid entirely and only 3 per cent were using the instrument with any degree of regularity. There is thus a need for counselling both on the issue of the aid and at intervals within the first few months of use regarding a number of matters. There include:

1   The construction of the aid and the purpose of the controls.
2   The limitations of a hearing aid, i.e. that it will not wholly provide the clear discrimination, selectivity and localisation of sound obtained from normal hearing.
3   Factors such as recruitment that may affect the benefit obtained.
4   Adjustment to the need to interpret many auditory signals against a background of increased sound.
5   The need to overcome any unwillingness to wear the aid in company because so doing indicates that the user has impaired hearing.

6   How to wear a body aid to the best advantage.
7   The maintenance of an aid and how to recognise minor faults.

Maintaining an aid

An aid will not function well if the batteries are leaking or wrongly inserted, or the ear-mould is blocked with wax. Batteries should always be of the type specified for the aid, correctly inserted and removed when spent or if the aid is not to be used for some time. Ear-moulds should be cleaned regularly in warm, soapy water using a pipe-cleaner to remove wax. The plastic tube on ear-level aids may eventually become stiff and break while the cords on body-worn aids also become brittle.

The checklist of possible faults in Table 10.1 may be useful.

The hearing therapist

In 1975 a report[6] of a sub-committee of the DHSS Advisory Committee on Services for Hearing Impaired People stated that the rehabilitation process started with the examination of the patient by an otologist and the fitting of a hearing aid. The report also recommended that a new class of worker known as a hearing therapist should be created within the NHS. The work of the hearing therapist begins where that of the PMT(A) ends. The main functions of the hearing therapist are to assess and so far as possible provide for medical, technical, social, financial, environmental, vocational and educational needs as part of the rehabilitative process. The hearing therapist will also help to maximise the patient's communication skills including the use of hearing aids and, where appropriate, supplementary instruction in speech-reading, auditory training and speech conservation. The range of activities of the hearing therapist who works as a member of a multi-displinary team which will also include clinical, technical and social work staff are shown in Fig. 10.3. In some areas the hearing therapist is augmented by voluntary workers who visit hearing impaired persons in their homes. Prior to taking up appointments, hearing therapists are required to take a one-year training course at the Centre for the Deaf of the City Literary Institute.

Table 10.1 Common hearing aid faults

Symptoms	Items to check	Possible fault	Action
Aid dead	Ear mould	Ear mould blocked with wax	Unclip from receiver and clean
	Batteries	Battery flat	Replace with new one
		Battery wrongly inserted	Insert correctly
		Contacts dirty or broken	Clean – with NHS aid this must be done at a hearing aid centre
	Plastic tube (on behind-the-ear aid)	Condensation in the tube	Remove ear mould and blow through the tube but *never into* the aid
	Cord (on body-worn aid)	Cord broken or intermittent	Replace cord
	Body of aid (on body-worn aid)	Faulty socket	Move cord in and out of socket. Return aid for repair
Low output from aid	Battery	Low voltage battery	Replace battery
	Volume control	Wrong setting of volume control	Correct setting
	Receiver	Faulty or wrong receiver	Replace receiver
Crackling	Cord or cord-plug socket (on body-worn aids)	Intermittent cord Faulty socket	Replace cord Return aid for repair
	Volume control	Dirty volume control	Clean volume control
Acoustic feedback	Ear mould	Poor fitting ear mould	Check fit of ear mould or replace

Environmental aids

Inability to hear the ringing of an alarm clock, doorbell or telephone; difficulty in communicating by telephone and the

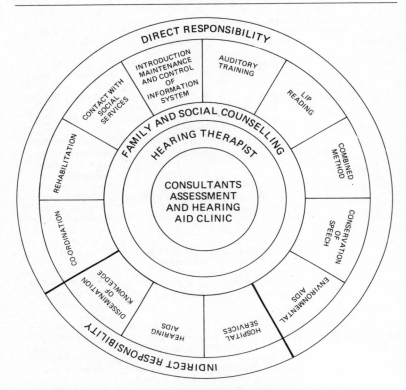

Fig. 10.3 Direct and indirect responsibilities of the hearing therapist

consciousness of causing inconvenience to others by turning up the volume of the television are some of the everyday problems encountered by hearing impaired persons. These problems may be overcome or minimised by the use of some ingenious environmental aids. Surveys have shown, however, that only a minority of persons who could be helped are aware of what is available. Other researchers reported that only 14 per cent of hearing aid users were aware of any environmental aids.[7] Another study stated that only 10 per cent of the sample of hearing impaired persons interviewed had any special aids and commented, 'The gap between respondents' knowledge about environmental aids and the possibilities presented by new technology is very wide indeed.'[8] This lack of knowledge is serious since, as Barcham and Stephens[9] discovered, 48 per cent of these respondents mentioned television/radio problems and 24 per cent and 20 per cent respectively difficulties with door and telephone bells.

An important aspect of the work of a hearing therapist is to bring appropriate environmental aids to the notice of potential users. Useful information regarding environmental aids and their suppliers can be obtained from the following publications: *Aids to Daily Living for the Hearing Impaired* (DHSS Ref STB/16/81); *Help for Handicapped People* available from British Telecom; the Report 'Help with Hearing' published in *WHICH*, October 1981 and the RNID booklet *Special Aids to Hearing*. The RNID has also published separate booklets including *TV/Radio Adaptors and the Loop System*. These aids are not free. The *Chronically Sick and Disabled Persons Act*, however, empowers a local authority, in approved cases, to provide such aids or give assistance towards their cost. The Manpower Services Commission may arrange for employers to have the permanent free loan of special aids to employment under its Job Introduction Scheme. Most environmental aids fall into one of three categories: alarm signals; telephone aids; television or radio aids.

Alarm signals

In a survey of hearing impaired persons in Blaby, Leicestershire, Skeikh and Verney[10] reported:

Many of the housewives described how they missed hearing doorbells, thus annoying tradesmen and missing friends. On the occasion when a caller was expected, they described how they would stay in the front room of the house in order to see him; much anxiety would have been saved by a flashing light door bell. One mother used to sit on the stairs in the hall when she was alone and her husband on night shift so she could hear the children if they cried.

Visual or other signals can reduce such tension. For hard of hearing people a low-frequency extension bell can be placed in the living room. People with a profounder loss may find it useful to install one of several types of light-flashing doorbells. These are mostly permanently installed, mains-powered units in which the pushing of the external door bell or, with one system, standing on a doormat, causes the house lighting to flash on or off or dim according to whether it is day or night. Using house lights has the disadvantages that electric clocks may be affected and some users may be averse at night-time to even momentary darkness. These drawbacks can be overcome by using special lamps to flash on and off.

Other light signals developed by the RNID are a flashing alarm clock and a baby alarm. In the former an electric alarm clock is modified to provide an outlet for a flashing mains supply into which a bedside lamp can be plugged. The lamp will continue to flash until the alarm is switched off.

With the baby alarm, noise picked up by a microphone on or near the child's cot causes a lamp to give a flashing signal. The sensitivity of the microphone can be adjusted to provide a threshold level below which the lamp will not be activated. Up to four extension lamps may be used to enable the warning to be seen in different rooms.

Where visual signals are inadequate or inappropriate, e.g. with deaf-blind persons, vibration can be used. A door warning system is available in which the pushing of the door bell activates a vibrator located in a portable receiver small enough to be slipped into the user's top pocket.

A vibrator alarm developed by the RNID also uses an electric alarm clock modified to provide a low voltage output to drive a large vibrator which can be placed under the pillow of a deaf person. At the set time the clock buzzes and the user will be aroused by powerful vibrations which continue until the alarm is cancelled. By linking the vibrator to a fire-warning detector, the RNID has devised a fire alarm system suitable for use in residential homes for profoundly deaf persons.

Telephone aids

British Telecom has the following range of aids to assist hard of hearing persons who experience difficulty in hearing the ringing of a telephone or hearing the caller.

Extension bells

These can be fitted in one or more rooms. Choice can be made from a range of bells of varying loudness including a 'cow gong' which has a more audible and distinctive note.

The Trimphone and Tone Ringer

The Trimphone, a modern handset, has a distinctive and

adjustable warbling tone heard more clearly than the standard telephone bell. The same tone is emitted by the Tone Ringer, an extension device for use with an ordinary telephone.

Visual signals

The simplest of these is a small neon lamp which glows in time with the ringing of the telephone bell. The lamp is fitted under a clear plastic cover in the back of the telephone handset.

Loudspeaking telephones

These remove the need to hold the telephone handset. If the loudspeaker switch is pressed the conversation can be heard by others who can check whether a hard of hearing person has heard aright. Speech from the loudspeakers may also be more easily heard by hearing aid users.

Amplifying handsets

With these the sound in the ear-piece can be increased by using a volume control on the side of the receiver to amplify the conversation to the required level.

Inductive couplers

An inductive coupler is a device which fits into the telephone handset to clarify incoming speech and eliminate background noise for wearers of hearing aids which incorporate a pick-up coil. All hearing aids with a 'T' (telephone) switch have a pick-up coil. British Telecom is in process of installing inductive couplers in all public call boxes. Kiosks already fitted display the special World Deaf symbol (Fig. 10.4).

The watch receiver

This is an extra earpiece which assists a hard of hearing person to listen to incoming speech with both ears and so reduce interference from other noises. The additional ear-piece can also be held against the microphone of some aids. This device is also useful to profoundly deaf persons since it enables someone with normal hearing to listen to incoming speech and repeat the message either in writing or so that it can be speech-read. The deaf person using the handset can then reply directly to the caller and in this way control the conversation.

Fig. 10.4 The World Deaf Symbol

Inter-communication devices for the profoundly deaf

It is certain that technological progress in the communication field will benefit the profoundly deaf. Because of the pace of such progress and the experimental nature of some projects, only three present applications are described.

Prestel

This is the computer-based information service developed by British Telecom. Information from the Prestel data base is fed by telephone line to a Prestel television set or an ordinary television fitted with an adaptor. Two deaf persons each with Prestel receivers fitted with alphanumeric keyboards can communicate by typing messages on their television screens. This is cheaper than the full Prestel service since users are charged only with the cost of the telephone call. The high cost of the equipment and the fact that typed messages take from four to six times as long as voice conversations so that deaf users have telephone bills much dearer than those of their hearing counterparts makes the use of this method of communication too expensive for most hearing impaired people.

Vistel

A cheaper device useful as a communication link only is the Deaf Communicating Terminal (DCT). A portable, battery-powered DCT weighing only 8 lb has been developed by the Breakthrough Trust in association with Kegwain Limited of Brighton under the name of Vistel (Visual Telephone). Vistel, which is a clear language soft-copy system comprises a typewriter keyboard and a small one-line display screen and can be used with any telephone handset other than a Trimphone. The Vistel can communicate with another Vistel, any other DCT using the British Telecom protocol or any Prestel set with a full alphanumeric keyboard. Calls are made by placing the telephone handset in the rubber cups at the rear of the unit and dialling the required number. The display screen indicates whether the number is ringing, or engaged. When contact is made the caller types out his message which will appear on the screens of both sender and receiver. Replies are sent and received in a similar manner. Vistel incorporates a memory and a facility known as 'Voice Over'. The memory serves three purposes. Emergency messages such as police, fire or ambulance can be stored as can messages typed in by the user for subsequent rapid transmission. Incoming messages can also be stored for the receiver to read at leisure. 'Voice Over' enables a deaf user with good speech to communicate easily with a hearing person. Using 'Voice Over', the deaf caller plugs in a headset and transmits his message vocally. Only the typed reply appears in the display screen. About 200 Vistel units were in current use in 1983.

Palantype transcription units

The first of these was developed by Dr Alan Newell, then of Southampton University, for the use of Jack Ashley, MP, at the House of Commons. The unit consists of a Palantype shorthand machine used for transcribing verbatim speech connected to a computer type display screen. Palantype script, phonetically-based and split into syllables is converted into a form which a deaf person can read after training. Mr Ashley sits in the House with his screen close by. The palantypist who acts as his 'ears' is located in the Press Gallery with the Palantype machine and electronic processing unit. While still in course of development the device has great potential for enabling deaf persons to follow lectures and meetings. An interesting experiment carried out by the RNID involved the establishment of a telephone bureau with a Palantype operator receiving calls and transmitting the speech of the hearing caller to a deaf person via Prestel. The BBC is also interested in using Palantype to provide live television subtitles.

Television and radio

Several devices enable hearing impaired persons to enjoy television and radio at an adequate volume without causing discomfort to others with normal hearing.

Headphones

Headphones for connection to radio, television or tape recorders can be obtained from most radio or hi-fi stores. Button ear-phones can be bought for radios.

The Varisond Radio Receiver is a battery-driven instrument which receives four VHF sound channels by pre-set buttons and has been specially designed for hard of hearing persons who might benefit from different sound levels and frequency settings for each ear. Output is to headphones each of which has its own controls. Sockets are provided for adapting to a record-player or tape-recorder microphone. In good reception areas, television sound can be picked up without connection to the television set.

Induction Loop Systems

These work in a similar way to inductive couplers. Induction loops can be connected to the loudspeaker terminals of the television. It is essential for safety reasons that this work is done by a qualified television engineer and that an isolating trans-former, matching the output of the set, is fitted between the set and the loop. A loop of ordinary household wire is then run round the room. Sound from the television may then be picked up by any number of hearing aids situated within the loop providing they have pick-up coils. One advantage is that the hearing aid user is not restricted to one position but can move freely about the room.

Adaptors

Essentially these devices designed to relay high volume sound from a television or radio directly to the user, comprise a control box with a connecting lead to the back of the set, an ear-piece and a cord. The control box, which can be placed on a chair-arm, houses a matching transformer, a volume control and other components. A range of adaptors is available, however, not all can be used with colour television sets.

Microphone aids

These units are small battery-powered amplifiers and function like hearing aids. A microphone is either attached to the loud-speaker grill or placed on a small table near the loudspeaker and connected to a hearing aid ear-piece by a long lead. An on/off switch and volume control is provided. When viewing, users of body-worn aids may find it useful to replace their normal lead by one say 12ft in length and to place the aid near the television loudspeaker.

Loop systems, adaptors and microphone aids assume that the user can hear speech. Those who, due to pre-lingual or profound acquired deafness lack this ability, can benefit from the use of Teletext and Viewdata and special services for deaf persons.

Teletext and Viewdata

Teletext services such as Ceefax and Orbit transmitted by the BBC and Oracle by ITV are one-way broadcast services sent out on the same transmission as conventional television pro-grammes. Viewdata and Prestel are two-way systems using telephone lines.

Teletext may assist deaf persons in three ways:
1   By providing pages of information which are updated some-times several times daily.
2   By special pages for the deaf such as *No need to shout* on Ceefax and *Earshot* on Oracle.
3   By subtitling some normal television programmes: details of programmes to be subtitled are given by the BBC on pp. 170 and 270 on Ceefax and Orbit respectively and p. 199 of Oracle.

Television receivers for Teletext are more expensive to buy or rent than standard sets without this facility. Once this expense has been met, however, the programmes are free. This is not so in the case of Prestel, which provides access to a vast store of information; the viewer is charged both for the telephone call to the local computer and the time connected to it. One advantage of Prestel is that deaf persons have access to the information provided without the need to contact strangers who may lack the willingness or patience to communicate verbally.

Other services

Television play synopses, available under a joint scheme run by the BBC and RNID, aim to provide sufficient information for hearing impaired persons to follow the plots of drama serials and one-off plays by prior reading. The synopses are only available for productions made by the BBC so that coverage is not available in respect of series brought in from American and other non-BBC services.

Interpreters using manual communication are provided for very few programmes such as Granada's *This is Your Right.*

Special programmes for the deaf including the children's programme *Vision On* have been transmitted. Overall, however, the time devoted to deaf viewers is a small proportion of that available. The Deaf Broadcasting Campaign has the aim of persuading at least one television organisation to broadcast a regular programme for the deaf including total communication and subtitles so that it can be viewed both by deaf and hearing persons.

Other environmental aids

Communicators

These are portable, battery-powered devices providing an amplified output to a pair of headphones fitted with ear-muffs. The frequency response is tailored to the requirements of the majority of hearing impairments, particularly those affecting elderly people. There is a separate hand-held microphone. Such units are useful for doctors, clergymen and others who wish to speak confidentially to a hearing impaired person.

The RNID Printator

This is a note pad with a smooth celluloid surface on which a message can be written with virtually any implement from a matchstick to a stylus. The message is erased when the celluloid surface is pulled out and pushed back in so that the device can be used repeatedly.

Obtaining environmental aids

The *WHICH* report of October 1981 contained the following useful advice:

When buying our samples – which we did as private individuals – we found that many firms were not really set up to deal with personal enquiries, expected to get orders only from local authorities, insisted on order numbers and so on. Usually there was not much sales literature around to enable you to see what you were buying. Rarely were we able to find shops stocking any of the aids and occasionally we had to wait several weeks for mail order products to come through. All in all, very unsatisfactory. If you have difficulty obtaining the aids you want and your local authority doesn't seem much help, ask the RNID or Hearing Aid Industry Association for lists of manufacturers.

References

1 Goldstein, M. A. *Problems of the Deaf*, Laryngoscope Press, St Louis, USA, 1933. Ch. 15, pp. 304–51.
2 Berger, K. W. and Millin, J. P. 'Hearing Aids' in Rose D. E. (Ed.), *Audiological Assessment*, Ch. 14, pp. 524–525.
3 Markides, Andreas. *The Aural Rehabilitation of Deafened Adults*, Scottish Association for the Deaf, 1976, p. 7.
4 McCall, R. F. *Hearing Loss – Hearing Aids*, South-East Regional Association for the Deaf, 1966, p. 18.
5 Brooks, Denzil N. 'Hearing Aid Candidates – Some Relevant Features', *British Journal of Audiology*, Vol. 13, 1979, pp. 81–84.
6 DHSS. *Report of a Sub-Comittee appointed to consider the Rehabilitation of the Adult Hearing Impaired*, September 1975, Para. 14.
7 Harris, M., Thomas, A. and Lamont, H. 'Deafness in Adults – Screening in General Practice', *Journal of the Royal College of Physicians*, March 1981, pp. 161–164.
8 Beattie, J. A. 'Social Aspects of Acquired Hearing loss in Adults', Unpublished PhD, Bradford, 1981.
9 Borcham and Stephens. *The Use of an Open-ended Problems Questionnaire in Auditory Rehabilitation*, p. 16.
10 Skeikh and Verney. *Report on the Survey of Hearing Impaired Persons in Blaby, Leicester, Leicestershire County Council, 1972.*

Chapter 11

Communication and auditory training

Communication, the process of passing information and under-standing from one person to another, has three elements: trans-mission, reception and comprehension. Thus, where no hearing impairment is present, speech and hearing are respectively the expressive and receptive elements. Communication does not take place, however, unless the person receiving the message has the knowledge or intelligence to comprehend the transmitted message. There are other ways of communicating that do not involve speech and hearing, such as writing and reading. Even where both hearing and vision are absent, we can still com-municate by tactile means as with the deaf-blind. Hearing loss, according to its severity and age of onset, is clearly a formidable barrier to normal communication. As shown in Chapters 5 and 8, pre-lingual hearing loss affects not only hearing but speech and the ability to comprehend many meanings.

We can, however, only communicate effectively if both sender and receiver use a common code or language and it is for this reason that in the education of deaf children the acquisition of a good command of the English language is of prime importance.

With deafened and hard of hearing persons it is the receptive element that is most affected since they experience most problems because of the inability to receive information from others through the medium of speech and from the environment in the form of sound.

Amplification, where appropriate, may, as indicated in Chapters 7 and 10, make it possible to exploit any residual hearing. The present chapter, however, is concerned with ways of facilitating communication through vision and listening, namely, speech-reading, manual communication, total communication and auditory training.

Speech-reading

Speech-reading has been defined as 'the art of understanding a speaker's thought by watching the movements of his mouth and facial expression'.[1] A more concise definition is that 'Speech-reading is the comprehension of spoken language through the medium of vision.'[2] Speech-reading is a more accurate term than lip-reading since the latter implies that only the lips are observed while, in fact, a speech-reader also observes tongue and jaw movements and, as recognised in the first of the above definitions, may also obtain valuable cues from the speaker's facial expression and body language.

Speech-reading may be utilised by the deaf, the deafened and the hard of hearing. With the pre-lingually deaf and the deafened, however, the hearing impairment is generally of such severity that even with the amplification to exploit any residual hearing they may largely abandon auditory cues to identify speech and rely wholly or mainly on vision to decode spoken messages. Conversely, the hard of hearing who can be helped to receive speech through the amplification provided by a hearing aid will regard speech-reading as a supplementary rather than an alternative method of enhancing their capacity to receive spoken communications.

The basis of speech-reading

Spoken language is composed of identifiable 'speech sounds' or phonemes. Phonemes have distinctive variations in air pressure that can be sensed by the air and can be divided into vowels and consonants. Vowels or 'resonated phonemes' provide the energy input of speech. Consonants or 'articulated sounds' make speech intelligible. The example below shows that by themselves vowels will never convey meaning. Consonants, however, can make a sentence intelligible even though the vowels are omitted.

Vowels: .. EA ... EE ... E ..... OU

consonants: Cl r sp ch g ts thr gh

In English there are about 40 speech sounds, which can be classified as shown in Table 11.1.

Table 11.1 English speech sounds
　　　　　Consonants (26)

Non-vocals (14) (Those with breath but no voice)	Vocals (12) (Those with voice)
h	.
wh	w
f	v
p	bm
t	dn
th (as in *thin*)	th (as in *though*)
s	z
sh	zh
ch	j
k	g ng
x = ks	.
q = kwh	.
.	r
.	l

Vowels (17)

Long vowels	Short vowels	Dipthongs
ar	oo	ou
aw	u	oi
oo	o	ie
oe	a	oe
er	e	ew
ee	i	

Table adapted from Burchett, J. H., *Lipreading*, 1965.

Some speech sounds, particularly *p*, *b*, *m*, *f*, *v*, *oo*, produced near the front of the mouth with maximum lip, tongue and jaw movements are clearly visible. Thus, in the list of speech sounds, *p*, *b* and *m* are grouped together because they are made by compressing the lips; *f* and *v* involve placing the lower lip against the top teeth; *oo* involves a marked rounding of the lips, while *sh* involves a combined protrusion and rounding of the lips. Tongue movements can be perceived in the placing of the tip of the tongue to the upper gum to form *t*, *d*, and *n*. Jaw movements also provide important cues in distinguishing between vowels: *ar* and *aw*, for example, are made with the mouth open as distinct from *i* in 'him' when the mouth is closed.

Only a proportion of speech sounds are visible and distinguishable. Those produced further back in the mouth with little movement of the lips, tongue or jaws, such as *k*, *g*, *h* and *v* cannot be seen on the lips. Although estimates vary, it is possible that up to 65 per cent of speech sounds cannot be seen and distinguished. As stated in the next section, this is only one of several problems that a speech-reader has to overcome.

The limitations of speech-reading

Many people think that speech-reading is a complete substitute for loss of hearing. Nothing could be further from the truth. Speech-reading has a number of limitations.

The usefulness of speech-reading is confined to speech. It offers no help with music, bird songs or warning signals. It is only of limited value in group conversation and is useless if the speaker is behind or out of the range of the speech-reader's vision.

As stated above, only a proportion of speech sounds are visible and distinguishable.

Speech sounds that look alike are called homophones. No speech-reader can distinguish between *p, b,* and *m,* since they involve the same lip movements.

There are also words, termed homophonous words, such as *pair* and *pear,* and *there* and *their,* which are visually the same. The only way in which the speech-reader can solve the problem is by relating the word to its context. A speech-reader has to choose the most appropriate word from *bending, pending* and *mending* to complete the sentence 'A court case is pending.'

The mouth is quicker than the eye. While in one second the average speaker makes from 13–15 articulatory movements, the eye of the receiver is capable of receiving only eight or nine such movements. For this reason alone the eye is going to miss a number of articulatory movements during each second of conversation. This loss is compounded by other factors. As mentioned earlier, a high proportion of speech sounds are invisible. The normal unit of conversation also tends to be the sentence rather than discrete words. The enquiry 'Are you going to town today?' is spoken as 'Areyougoingtotowntoday?' Unless there is a visible pause between each word, the speech-reader has to cope with a flowing series of movements of varying degrees of visibility.

Environmental factors such as lighting and distance also pose problems for the speech-reader. Obviously it is not possible to speech-read in the dark. The pupils of a speech-reader's eyes are constricted if he has to look into a light source situated behind the speaker. While, with normal vision it is possible to speech-read at distances of up to 24ft, it is easier to do so at normal conversational distances: about 5ft is probably the ideal distance.

Speakers vary in the ease with which they can be speech-read. In general, it is harder for a speech-reader to comprehend a stranger than someone who is familiar. As indicated, speech-reading increases in difficulty with the rapidity of the speaker's delivery. Speakers with expressive faces are easier to speech-read than the converse. Speakers who look away, put their hands over their mouths, or smoke cigarettes or pipes while speaking pose problems for speech-readers. Beards and moustaches may also present difficulties. From the above certain characteristics of speech-reading can be identified.

1   Even for highly accomplished practitioners, speech-reading involves a considerable element of educated guesswork.
2   Speech-reading, like reading or the hearing of speech, is not a process which endeavours to identify individual words or articulatory movements. Speech-reading is a *total* process, the aim being to comprehend the essential thought that is being communicated. In doing this, the speech-reader will be alert to contextual and environmental cues, such as key words, the subject under discussion, the environment in which the message is being received, and the gestures and facial expressions of the speaker.
3   Speech-reading requires intense concentration and fatigue may cause the speech-reader's attention to wander.

The Sympathetic Hearing Scheme has been introduced to help deaf and hard of hearing people to lead easier lives. The scheme utilises the World Deaf Symbol shown on page 136 and eventually it is hoped that the symbol will be displayed wherever someone is available to serve a deaf or hard of hearing person on request. The following guidelines have been prepared to assist anyone dealing with a hearing impaired person:

1   Do *not* shout. It is a common reaction, but it does not help and only causes embarrassment.
2   Speak slowly and clearly, but do not exaggerate your facial movements or distort your face.
3   Try to face the light as well as the person you are speaking to.
4   Cut out as much background noise as possible.
5   Do not smoke, eat or do anything else that involves putting

your hand in front of your face. Lip readers must be able to see your mouth.

6 Use plain language. Many words look the same to lip readers. The more common the word the better.

7 If you are not immediately understood, try rephrasing what you are saying.

8 Write things down if you think it is necessary. Again it is easier for you both if you use common and quite short words.

9 If a deaf customer is accompanied by a hearing friend, address what you are saying to the customer. The friend will still be able to follow and help if needed.

The advantages of speech-reading

In the light of the above limitations, Hutton's[3] opinion that visual cues alone are unlikely to provide sufficient information for effective communication is hardly surprising. Speech-reading is of great importance, however, particularly when it is part of a multisensory approach to aural rehabilitation. Thus, competency in speech-reading as a component of the oral approach to the education of hearing impaired children is more likely to be acquired when residual hearing can be exploited by appropriate amplification. With both children and adults there are numerous reasons why speech-reading used in conjunction with a hearing aid can help to cancel out the limitations of an exclusive reliance on either vision or hearing. Speech-reading can help to overcome discrimination difficulties experienced in the use of an aid particularly in cases of sensorineural loss where a hearing aid user may have problems with distortion and recruitment. Some high frequency speech sounds can easily be distinguished visually. McCall[4] points out that

Those with severe deafness will find lip-reading (speech-reading) easier if an aid can provide any sound, even rhythm of voice. Used with memory of normal sound of speech, lipreading can give the effect of 'hearing' the voice throughout.

Speech-reading can also provide considerable psychological support. It provides increased confidence in social situations. Hearing aid users know that they will not be completely helpless should their instrument let them down. Especially with traumatically deafened persons, where immediate measures to overcome depression are essential, speech-reading can offer a lifeline both in the effort required to achieve proficiency, which, to some extent, can counteract brooding, and the promise it gives of being able to maintain contact with hearing people. Speech-reading may be beneficial even in cases of mild hearing loss which do not warrant the use of an aid. It is particularly important in cases of sensorineural or mixed sensorineural loss; conductive loss that cannot be treated by surgery or when surgery is not acceptable; where the degree of loss is 70 dB or greater over the speech frequencies; and where the usefulness of an aid is reduced by discrimination difficulties.

Learning to speech-read

Speech-reading is best learned in a class situation. Local education authorities will usually provide tuition at a further education college if sufficient persons can be found to form a speech-reading class. Where there is difficulty in obtaining tuition, an approach should be made to the RNID or BAHOH.

Most teachers of speech-reading combine both analytical or synthetical elements in a speech-reading lesson. The aim of the analytical element is to train the eyes of the pupil to recognise speech sounds visually. The purpose of the synthetical element is to train the mind to grasp the total impact of the message even though individual words are not recognised.

Speech-reading is a skill. As with other skills, performers are likely to differ in their aptitude and performance. Although a number of tests have been devised to predict aptitude for speech-reading and the effectiveness of performance, these have not been satisfactorily validated, and they are largely un-standardised. Empirically, it appears that motivation and persistence are more important in a would-be speech-reader than intelligence, although the latter, involving the capacity to see relationships, is not unimportant.

Fusfield[5], in a study of effectiveness in speech-reading, obtained the views of two groups of hearing impaired persons – one group comprised expert speech-readers; the second those who experience great difficulty with speech-reading. Among his findings were the following:

1   There are good lipreaders, some expert to a high degree. There are others of the same general intelligence contour, for whom the skill is either non-existent or present only in an indifferent manner.
2   Some good lipreaders have the tendency when familiar with the

threads of a conversation to 'think ahead', i.e. to anticipate. This practice, however, can be unreliable.

3 Good lipreaders are alert to their general environment.
4 Natural talent for lipreading is not necessarily the same as high intelligence, but a special aptitude similar to trait combinations, which make for success in music, art or mechanical skill.
5 No single factor fully accounts for lipreading efficiency but rather a combination of circumstances – natural aptitude, easy command of the English language, acquaintance with the vagaries present in speech, and a large functioning vocabulary.
6 One common denominator was present in all skilled lipreaders. This was a personality make-up that did not shake under initial failure, or was not 'floored' when things went wrong lipreading-wise. Thus, invariably, if the lipreader did not immediately 'catch on', the reaction was 'Beg pardon?', or 'I'm sorry, I didn't get you' – so inviting repetition with greater care.

Manual communication

Manual communication is a general term for the visual transmission of information by pictorial or ideagraphical representations produced by the hands, arms, face and body. It is not easy to categorise the various systems of manual communication without overlapping. One possible, but not exhaustive, classification is as follows:
1 Finger-spelling.
2 Manual systems based on English language usage, e.g. Signed English; The Paget-Gorman Sign System.
3 Manual systems complementary to speech-reading, e.g. The Danish Mouth-hand System; Cued Speech.
4 British Sign Language.
5 International sign language, e.g. Gestuno.

Finger-spelling

As shown by Fig. 11.1, finger-spelling simply involves positioning the fingers in 26 different positions to represent the 26 letters of the alphabet. The five vowels are indicated by touching with the right forefinger, the tip of the left thumb for *A*, the first finger for *E*, the middle one for *I*, the next for *O* and the little finger for *U*. For the consonants, the position of the fingers roughly forms the shape of the printed letter.

Finger-spelling can be used in conjunction with speech, speech-reading, amplification and with other manual methods.

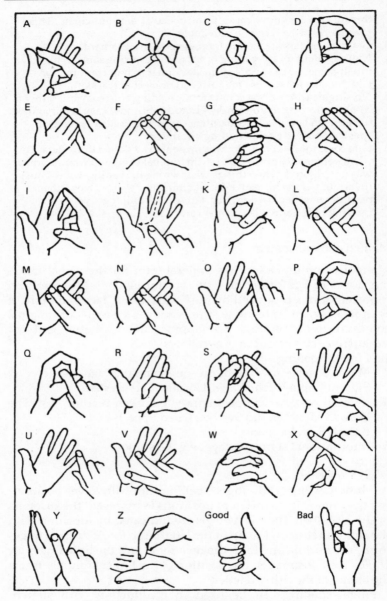

Fig. 11.1 The manual alphabet, English system

It is especially useful for spelling out proper names, foreign or unusual words and in manual communication, where there is no sign.

Finger-spelling can be quickly learned but regular practice over a considerable time is needed before rapid finger-spelling can be read. When this proficiency has been attained, finger-spelling is about twice as rapid as writing. The RNID has produced a version of the popular crossword game *Kan-U-Go* to provide a pleasant way of achieving proficiency with finger-spelling.

Since finger-spelling is the easiest means of communicating with severely hearing impaired persons, the following hints are given:

1 Hold the left hand with the palm towards the person being addressed.
2 Keep the fingers of the left hand outspread, making them easier to see.
3 Normally, the finger-speller does not pause for punctuation or capitals; words run together with a space between them. At first, however, it is easier to read if the finger-speller makes a break at the end of each word.
4 Special care is needed with vowels since the wrong touch of a vowel finger can completely alter a word, e.g. *bear* to *beer*.

Manual systems based on English language usage

Signed English. In this system ordinary grammatical English is translated into British Sign Language (BSL) by means of finger-spelling or other non-verbal forms of communication. As Montgomery points out.[6]

Some forms of Signed English use special signs to indicate grammatical features such as tense, plurality and gender which are not always apparent in BSL. New signs such as those for 'the', 'sentence' and 'paragraph' have been invented to maintain the parallel between spoken, written and signed forms of English. Some have even made up signs for punctuation marks. . . .

The Paget-Gorman Systematic Sign System. This system was pioneered by Sir Richard Paget and developed by Dr Pierre Gorman, a former librarian of the RNID, and Lady Paget. It aims to help hearing impaired children to acquire at an early age an understanding of correct language in association with speech and speech-reading. It can also assist hearing persons whose language has been inadequately developed by other methods of teaching. The system includes an extensive vocabulary of carefully derived signs intended to be used in conjunction with speech. This vocabulary can be further extended by signed affixes which, *inter alia,* indicate plurality in nouns, the comparative and superlative forms of adjectives, the past tense and passive mood of verbs and such suffixes as *ing, ly* and *y.* Distinct signs are used for all parts of the verb *to be,* and all pronouns. Punctuation marks may be signed where required for teaching purposes.

Although the only examples of a systematic sign language with a normal grammatical structure reported to the Lewis Committee,[7] Paget-Gorman is not without its disadvantages. These, summarised by Denmark,[8] are that it is not used by the prelingually deaf population; only few professional workers are conversant with the method; it is more difficult to learn than BSL; too difficult to learn for the child of limited potential and that it does not enable the deaf child who uses the method to integrate into the deaf community.

Manual systems complementary to speech-reading

Two systems are extant, the Danish Mouth-hand system, and Cued Speech. Both aim to increase the accuracy of speech-reading and reduce the strain involved by enabling speech sounds to be more easily recognised. These systems are particularly useful with traumatically deafened persons, or where at least one member of a family has a severe hearing loss which cannot be overcome with a hearing aid.

The Danish Mouth-hand System. This was devised in 1902 by Georg Forchhammar, a Danish teacher of the deaf. Forchhammar recognised that only 30 per cent of all Danish speech sounds could be identified with reasonable certainty. As the vowels belonged to this 30 per cent, it was clear that the main difficulties lay with the consonants. As stated earlier, the sounds *p, b* and *m* are identical on the lips and the correct word has to be determined from the context in which it is used. In the English version of Forchhammar's system, 18 symbols are used to represent 22 consonant sounds. Separate symbols are provided for *p, b* and *m* so that guesswork is eliminated.

As shown in Fig. 11.2, the various movements are made by one hand positioned under the chin and close to the chest of the

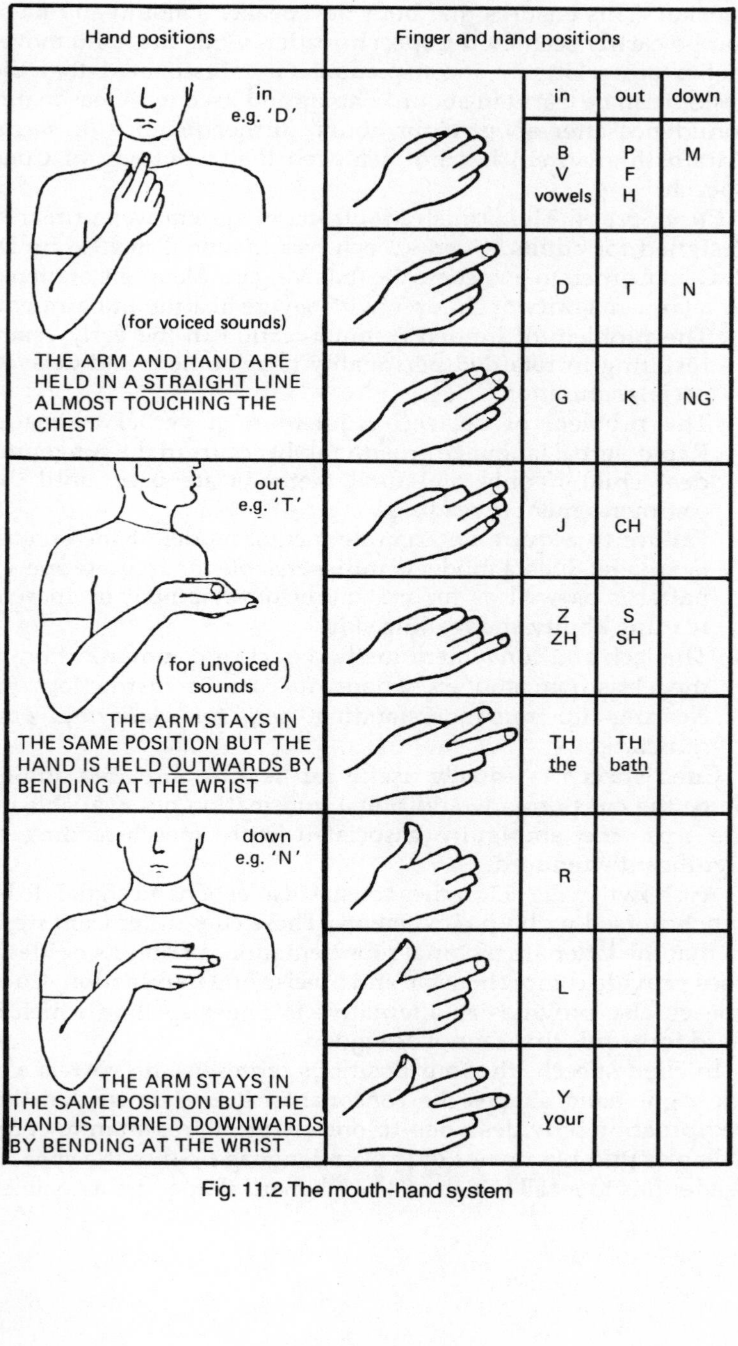

Hand positions	Finger and hand positions			
		in	out	down
in e.g. 'D' (for voiced sounds) THE ARM AND HAND ARE HELD IN A <u>STRAIGHT</u> LINE ALMOST TOUCHING THE CHEST		B V vowels	P F H	M
		D	T	N
		G	K	NG
out e.g. 'T' (for unvoiced) sounds THE ARM STAYS IN THE SAME POSITION BUT THE HAND IS HELD <u>OUTWARDS</u> BY BENDING AT THE WRIST		J	CH	
		Z ZH	S SH	
		TH <u>the</u>	TH ba<u>th</u>	
down e.g. 'N' THE ARM STAYS IN THE SAME POSITION BUT THE HAND IS TURNED <u>DOWNWARDS</u> BY BENDING AT THE WRIST		R		
		L		
		Y <u>y</u>our		

Fig. 11.2 The mouth-hand system

speaker. This ensures that both the speaker's mouth and hand can be clearly seen by the speech-reader, while the hand movements are relatively inconspicuous. It is estimated that the system can be learnt in about 12 hours and used with reasonable confidence after about eight hours' further practice. In Great Britain this system has not achieved the popularity of Cued Speech.

Cued Speech. The Danish Mouth-hand system was primarily designed for adults. Cued speech was invented in 1966 by Dr R. Orin Cornett to overcome the following problems encountered by a large majority of children with severe hearing impairment:

1   The problem of limited communication in the early years, resulting in retarded personality development and delayed social maturation.
2   The problem of delayed acquisition of verbal language. Rapid verbal language growth rarely occurs in the congenital deaf child if only oral-aural methods are used until the commencement of reading.
3   Failure to acquire an accurate mental model of the spoken language. Such a model is indispensable for accurate speech patterns as well as for maximum development of speech-reading ability and reading skill.
4   The lack of a convenient method of clear communication in the classroom and elsewhere, for use in instruction, for clearing up misunderstanding and for clarifying pronunciation.

Cued speech is equally useful for hearing impaired adults. Since the cues provide additional information not available on the lips, the ambiguity associated with speech-reading is significantly reduced.

As shown in Fig. 11.3, cues consist of a set of hand signals to be synchronised with lip movements. These cues differ from signs in that the latter are pictorial representations of objects or ideas; cues provide comprehensive and precise oral information. Cued speech also provides an alternative to finger-spelling which is used for words that cannot be signed.

In cued speech, the four positions represent the vowels and the right hand shapes the consonants. It is claimed that this combination provides a one-to-one visible representation of the syllables and phonemes of spoken language. Since the speech-reader has to recall which of 24 consonant shapes are associated

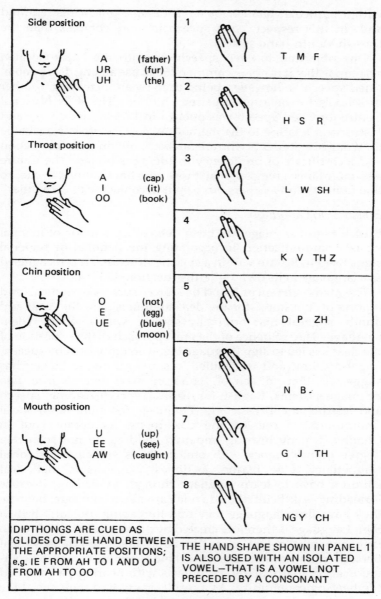

Fig. 11.3 Cued speech

with a particular handshape, considerable practice is required and, in this respect, cued speech is more complex than the Danish Mouth-hand system.

One objection to cued speech, as with the Paget-Gorman system, is that it is not in common social use among deaf people. Cued speech is, however, being used by an increasing number of schools for hearing impaired children. The Kids National Centre for Cued Speech was opened in 1975 to give advice and instruction relating to the method. A postal course is available for would-be students who are unable to obtain class instruction and a certificate of proficiency in cueing is issued. The Centre also maintains a register of all those who have learned to cue, so that families and teachers can be put in contact with each other.

British Sign Language

British Sign Language has been defined as 'a mode of manual visual communication incorporating the national or regional signs used in Britain within a specific structure'. It is recognised as a language in its own right, distinct from English.[9]

The many references found in sources such as periodicals and reports of 'missions' for the deaf to 'mutes' and the 'deaf and dumb' suggest that originally signing was a wholly silent language. The influence of the oral approach to the education of the deaf has led to sign language being accompanied by speech, finger-spelling and uncodified gestures or signs. Stelle[10] has suggested that in school, children may diverge into two language systems, English for reading, speech-reading, speech and lessons and British Sign Language for more rapid social communication outside the class-room. As pointed out in Chapter 7 many hearing impaired children do not achieve a degree of proficiency with oral methods sufficient for social competency. One reason, as Jones[11] suggests is that 'deaf children have to learn language through lipreading; because lipreading is difficult, they do not learn much language; because they have little language they find lipreading difficult'. British Sign Language is therefore created by those who have little or no language in the first place. In adult life, pre-lingually deaf persons may have to use other, more taxing means of communication, particularly in contacts with hearing persons and the hearing community. As a result, many find their social life within the welfare societies for the adult deaf, possibly because in such a community they are 'normal' and have opportunities for the achievement of self-esteem and communication without strain through the language of signs.

Signs may be classified into several categories. *Natural* signs may have some analogy to the idea suggested but not described, e.g. head resting on palms together, for 'go to sleep'. *Derivative* signs may be developed from some root idea such as the sign for girl or woman, where the upright forefinger is moved across the mouth to convey the idea of a beardless person. In contrast the sign for man is made by bringing the first down the face to indicate a beard. *Indicative* signs are made by pointing to the object intended. Some signs such as thumbs up for 'good' have no analogous associations. The number of signs in use is limited and words for which no signs exist must be finger-spelled. The RNID publishes a book, *Sign and Say* which illustrates many British signs. The BDA also published *The Language of the Silent World* (now out of print). A definitive dictionary of British Sign Language is also in the course of preparation by the BDA.

BSL is not standardised and signs have many regional variations. It is ungrammatical and tends to follow the order in which ideas are generated with the most important or dominant concept coming first; thus, the sentence 'I am going shopping' would be converted to 'shopping I go'. BSL is not a written language and is not codified. It is of only limited use for technical or academic purposes but is excellent for personal conversation.

Deuchars[12] distinguishes between 'High' and 'Low' forms of sign language. Both use the vocabulary of BSL but 'High' is based on English and is essentially Signed English. With 'Low', the rules of syntax are disregarded. The variety of signing used probably depends on the needs of the individual deaf person. Gorman[13] identified four categories of deaf persons requiring interpretation:

1 The better educated who needs a literal translation.
2 The average with poor linguistic and vocabulary attainment.
3 The dull and backward.
4 The mentally defective or uneducated.

From the standpoint of signing the needs of the first three categories are met respectively by Signed English; BSL; and BSL used less fluently.

The fourth category may benefit from the *Makaton Vocabulary* which has been specially designed to provide a controlled method of teaching BSL to mentally handicapped children and adults. Details of this approach can be obtained from the Makaton Vocabulary Development Project.

International Sign Language

Gestuno is the sign language created by the World Federation of the Deaf for use at international conferences and meetings of deaf people. It therefore performs the same function for national sign languages as Esperanto does for auditory language. In 1975 the BDA produced a photographic dictionary of Gestuno which has achieved international circulation.

Learning manual communication

As with speech-reading classes, manual communcation can be provided by a local education authority where it can be shown that a sufficient number of persons wish a class to be provided. As stated in Chapter 8, the Council for the Advancement of Communication with Deaf People is concerned with the establishment of schemes of training and certification on a local regional and national basis.

Total communication

The most comprehensive definition of total communication is that adopted by the Maryland School for the Deaf in 1970:

Total Communication is the right of every child to learn to use all forms of communication so that he may have competence at the earliest possible age. This implies introduction to a reliable, receptive, expressive symbol system in the pre-school years between the ages of one and five. Total communication includes the full spectrum of language modes: child-devised gestures, formal sign language, speech, speech reading, finger spelling, reading and writing. Every deaf child has the opportunity to develop any remnant of residual hearing for the enhancement of speech and speech reading skills through the use of individual and/or fidelity group amplification systems.

Conrad[14] has defined total communication more narrowly as 'manually aided oral communication'. On this basis total communication is little more than a development of the combined method or 'Siglish' in which signs and finger-spelling are used to supplement communication by speech and speech-reading. Total communication, however, is predominantly a philosophy rather than a method, and is often contrasted with the 'Limited Communication Approach' such as pure oralism.

While support for total communication is found among some educators, particularly in the USA, the main British advocates are those working with adult pre-lingually deaf persons. Vernon[15] makes the following statements in support of it:

1   The deaf pre-school child is provided from the start with a language environment.

2   The approach assists rather than hinders the development of language and communication skills such as speech and speech-reading.

3   Hearing parents have a greater potential for helping a deaf child when total communication is used.

4   The integration of a deaf child into hearing society is assisted and adjustment to hearing people is fostered.

5   Total communication is supported by psychiatrists who have worked extensively in the field of hearing impairment.

6   Total communication is also supported by the overwhelming majority of pre-lingually deaf persons including those who have been taught by oral methods.

7   Sign language is more than a language in the linguistic sense. It is also a means of expressing emotion.

Workers with the adult deaf have suggested some additional reasons in favour of total communication:

8   The limited vocabulary and lack of fluency in the use of idiomatic English which is characteristic of many pre-lingually deaf persons adversely affects speech-reading ability.

9   Signing is a 'natural' communication method for the deaf and requires no special learning effort.

10   Total communication, utilising several approaches, is more certain than speech and speech-reading alone and is more useful in adult life when a deaf person has to comprehend a message accurately as in medical and legal situations.

11   Total communication, including signs and finger-spelling, is the only practicable way in which school assemblies, religious services, dramatic presentations and public meetings can be communicated to groups of deaf persons.

12   Signs and finger-spelling impose less strain on the eyes and minds of deaf persons than where speech and speech-reading are exclusively used.

Conrad[16] has stated that to his knowledge there is not 'in English' a single published account which sets out the outcome, the achievements and the shortcomings of a good oral education. The main arguments against total communication are that the inclusion of non-linguistic means of communication adversely affects linguistic development; that the use of signs is a disincentive to speak, speech-read and listen, and that, the greater the competency of a deaf person in oral communication, the easier it will be to integrate into hearing society.

The Lewis Committee recognised that there was general agreement that the principal aims in educating hearing impaired children should be 'to enable them to realise their full potential and so far as possible take their place in society in due course as literate adults with whole personalities which they can express through generally understood media of communication'.[17] The same Report also stated that almost unanimously there was no wish for a return to the education by wholly silent methods nor any witnesses who claimed that 'Exclusively oral methods are appropriate for all deaf children at all stages of education; but it was generally agreed that there are stages at which oral methods alone are likely to produce the most satisfactory results irrespective of the aptitudes and characteristics of individual children.'[18] The main area of contention is whether from the start total communication, in which signs and finger-spelling are used to supplement oral/aural methods, can be used without detriment to the linguistic development of the deaf child and his or her capacity to integrate into the hearing world.

The Lewis Committee also stressed the need for research studies to determine whether or not and in what circumstances the introduction of manual media of communication would lead to improvement in the education of deaf children.[19] This is commendable but a warning by Nix[20] who reviewed 17 research studies frequently cited in support of total communication deserves attention.

The finding of the studies have been misinterpreted and inappropriately generalised beyond the children examined and the public residential school setting, even though some of the investigators specifically cautioned against this.

Meanwhile Jordan[21] reported in 1981 that, in UK schools, changes from oral to total communication is taking place at an increasing rate with total communication being more wide-spread in Scottish than English schools.

Auditory training

Carhart[22] has defined auditory training as 'the process of teaching the child or adult who is hard of hearing to take full advantage of the sound clues which are still available to him'. Some writers take a wider view of auditory training to encompass also the provision of hearing aids, speech-reading, conversation and counselling although procedures such as hearing aid fitting, speech training and conversation are allied to, rather than included in, auditory training. The aims of auditory training differ with children and adults.

Children

Boothroyd[23] has stated that with children the aim is to 'provide contrived exieriences through which hearing impaired children develop auditory skills that other children obtain naturally'. Carhart[22] identified four stages in this skill development. The first stage involves directing the child's attention to sound so that noises are recognised as meaningful. The next stage, that of gross discrimination, aims at training the child to distinguish between highly dissimilar noises such as those produced by drums, cymbals and car horns. The penultimate stage seeks to help the child to discriminate broadly among simple speech patterns including vowels and familiar meaningful phrases, e.g. 'Do you want a drink?' The final stage aims at developing precise discrimination for speech including the acquisition of a large vocabulary and the ability to follow connected discourse. Developments in the use of amplification and later work in the field of aural rehabilitation have modified the Carhart approach. With the early exploitation of residual hearing by amplification the need to develop an awareness of sound is of less importance. Approaches to auditory training developed by other workers in this field reflect the advances that have taken place in the early detection of hearing impairment and an increased emphasis in integrating measures for improving the auditory perception of speech with other educational procedures rather than treating them as separate activities.

Adults

With children the aim is the recognition and use of auditory cues. With adults, as Carhart points out, 'the task is primarily one of re-educating an impaired ability. The person must become fully aware of his limitations in discrimination and must get accustomed once more to hearing loud sounds, distinguishing speech from noise and so forth.' Persons with a significant hearing loss tend to listen selectively thereby giving the impression that they can 'hear when they want to'. It is not often understood that the tension and anxiety experienced by a hearing impaired person is very fatiguing and that such selective listening is a conscious or unconscious way of conserving energy. Elderly persons often find difficulty in adjusting to the unwanted ambient noise that accompanies the use of a hearing aid and find relief in withdrawing into a world of silence. If habitual inattention is to be counteracted it is necessary, as Carhart says, that an attitude of 'critical listening' should be established from the outset. Auditory training which can increase the consciousness of environmental sound and improve speech discrimination may assist adults to obtain the maximum benefit from a hearing aid. It may also result in an enhanced awareness of listening behaviour thereby avoiding some annoyance to others because of inattention.

Factors in auditory training

Whether an individual person will benefit from auditory training depends on both general and specific factors. General factors include data obtained from audiometric tests for pure-tones and speech, the cause, nature and extent of the hearing loss; the age of onset and the degree of impairment. Probably the best rough and ready indication for or against auditory training is the ability to discriminate between speech sounds.

Markides[24] has identified four groups of specific factors that influence the effectiveness of auditory training: availability of services; the hearing impaired person and his family; the methods followed; and the equipment used. In relation to 'the hearing impaired person and his family', Markides rightly states that auditory training involves systematic and persistent practice under the direction of a professional therapist with the end result depending primarily on the qualities of the therapist combined with attributes relating to the individual hearing impaired person, including motivation; co-operation with the therapist; age; intelligence; systematic practice; habituation; understanding of the basic principles involved and the degree, pattern and type of hearing impairment.

One important factor is that of what criteria should be used to evaluate the effectiveness of auditory training. Bamford[25] has stated that traditionally auditory discrimination tests, various speech and language tests, localisation tests and measures of auditory handicap and social adjustment have been used as well as (for children) general attainment tests. At the end of a perceptive paper, Bamford concludes that well-designed studies of the effectiveness of auditory training are the exception and 'It remains true that we do not understand why some children and adults appararently respond to auditory training and others do not.'

Facilities for auditory training

Although it is likely that the facilities for auditory training will improve as the number of hearing therapists in post increases, the provision of such training at the time of writing is at the best 'patchy' and in some areas non-existent. An individual should first ascertain through his otologist, audiological physician or audiologist whether he would be likely to benefit from auditory training. If auditory training would be beneficial, but no facilities are available locally, the matter might be raised with the health authority, the social services department of the local authority in which the enquirer resides or with the RNID or BAHOH.

References

1 Jeffers, J. and Bailey, M. *Speech Reading*, Charles C. Thomas, Springfield (III), 1971.
2 American Hearing Society. *Hearing Loss a Community Loss*, 1958, p. 70.
3 Hutton, C. 'Combining Auditory and Visual Stimuli in Aural Rehabilitation, *Volta Review*, Vol. 61, 1959, pp. 316–319.
4 McCall, R. F. *Hearing Loss – Hearing Aids*, South-East Regional Association for the Deaf, 1966, p. 22.
5 Fusfield, I. S. 'Factors in Lipreading as Determined by the Lipreader, *American Annals of the Deaf*, March 1958, pp. 234–237.

6   Montgomery, G. 'Alien Communication. Sign Systems Extant in the U.K.', *Supplement to the British Deaf News*, March/April 1981.
7   *The Education of Deaf Children, Report of the Lewis Committee*, HMSO 1964, para. 32(c), p. 19.
8   Denmark, J. 'Methods of Communication in the Education of Deaf Children, *Methods of Communication Currently used in the Education of Deaf Children*, RNID 1975, p. 76.
9   British Association of Teachers of the Deaf. *Teacher of the Deaf*, July 1980, pp. 4–5.
10 Stelle, T. W. *A Primer for Parents with Deaf Children*, Scottish Workshop Publications, 1980.
11 Jones, K. D. *The Adult Deaf Population of South Humberside*, unpublished M Phil thesis, University of Nottingham, 1983.
12 Deuchars, M. *Diglossia in Britain Sign Language*, unpublished PhD thesis, Stanford University, 1978, p. 9.
13 Gorman, P. P. *Certain Social and Psychological Difficulties Facing the Deaf Person in the English Community*, unpublished PhD thesis, Cambridge, 1960, pp. 219–220.
14 Conrad, R. *Matters Arising in Methods of Communication Currently Used in the Education of Deaf Children*, RNID, 1976, p. 147.
15 Vernon, M. *Total Communication in Spotlight on Communication*, Papers given at the BDA Congress, 1974.
16 Conrad, R. as (14) above p. 148.
17 *The Education of Deaf Children, Report of the Lewis Committee*, HMSO, 1968, para. 273.
18 Ibid. para. 274.
19 Ibid. para. 294.
20 Nix, G. W. 'Total Communication. A Review of the Studies Offered in the Support.' *Volta Review* No. 77, November 1975, p. 493.
21 Jordan, I. K. 'Communication Methods used at Schools for the Deaf and Partially Hearing and at Units for Partially Hearing Children in the United Kingdom, *Surdometrika*, Vol. III, No. 11, June 1981, p. 4.
22 Carhart, R. 'Auditory Training', Davis H. (Ed.), *Hearing and Deafness*, Murray Hill Books, 1947, Ch. 10. p. 282.
23 Boothroyd, A. 'Discrimination by Partially Hearing Children of Frequency Distorted Speech, *Audiology*, Vol. 6, 1967, pp. 136–145.
24 Markides, A. 'Rehabilitation of People with Acquired Deafness in Adulthood', *British Journal of Audiology, Supplement No. 1*, March 1977.
25 Bamford, J. 'Auditory Training – What is it, what is it supposed to do, and does it do it?, *British Journal of Audiology*, Vol. 15, 1981, pp. 75–78.

Chapter 12

Statutory and voluntary provision for the hearing impaired

Both statutory and voluntary agencies are concerned with hearing impairment. This chapter aims to outline the available provision.

Statutory provision

Statutory provision of importance to hearing impaired persons relates to hearing aids, education, employment, health, social security and the social services.

Hearing aids

The Hearing Aid Council Act 1968 is the only statute exclusively concerned with hearing impairment. The Act provides for the establishment of a Hearing Aid Council, the registration and training of suppliers of aids and the regulation of trade practices including the establishment of procedures for investigating complaints by a Disciplinary Committee comprising Council members. For the purpose of the Act a dispenser of hearing aids is defined as:

An individual who conducts or seeks to conduct oral negotiations with a view to effecting the supply of a hearing aid, whether by him or another, to or for the use of a person with impaired hearing.

Education

The education of hearing impaired children is still based on the Education Act 1944 which places a duty on every local education authority to provide schools sufficient in number, character and equipment to afford all pupils opportunities for education offer-

165

ing such variety of instruction and training as may be desirable in view of their different ages, abilities and aptitudes, and of the different periods for which they may be expected to remain at school.

The 1944 Act did not mention any specific disability but provided that the Minister should 'make Regulations defining the several categories of pupils requiring special educational treatment and making provisions as to the special methods appropriate for the education of each category'. This section of the Act was implemented by Regulations, first issued in 1945, which specified ten classes of handicapped pupils including the deaf and partially deaf. In 1962 the 'partially deaf' became the 'partially hearing'.

As stated in Chapter 7, the Education Act 1981 replaced the ten classes of handicapped pupils and laid down that special educational provision should be based on the special education needs of individual children. Under the general provisions for further education a local education authority has discretionary powers to provide special classes. These may, for example, include speech-reading or instruction in manual communication.

Employment

The Disabled Persons Employment Acts, 1944 and 1958 aim to assist those handicapped by some form of disability to obtain and retain 'employment suitable to their capacities which utilises their skill to the best advantage'. A disabled person is defined as 'one who on account of injury, disease or congenital deformity is substantially handicapped in obtaining or keeping suitable employment'. An outline of the help available to hearing impaired people under these Acts is given in Chapter 8.

Health

The National Health Service Act 1946 laid upon the then Minister of Health a duty to 'promote the establishment of a comprehensive health service . . . designed to secure improvement in the physical and mental health of the people . . . and the prevention, diagnosis and treatment of illness and for that purpose to provide or ensure the provision of services in accordance with . . . the Act'. The Ministry of Health was merged with the Department of Health and Social Security on 1 November 1968. By the National Health Services Re-organisation Act

1973 the School Health Service became part of the NHS.

Preventive medicine such as rubella vaccination has an important role in preventing hearing impairment. The Abortion Act 1967 provides that the termination of pregnancy is no longer a criminal offence if in the opinion of two medical practitioners there is a substantial risk that if the child were born it would suffer from such physical or mental abnormalities as to be seriously handicapped. In 1979 and 1980, the DHSS issued circulars urging area health authorities to intensify the vaccination programme against congenital rubella.

The provisions for the screening for hearing impairment of pre-school and school children were described in Chapter 4.

The general practitioner and hospital and specialist services administered under the Act provide for diagnosis and treatment of all conditions including hearing impairment.

In 1943, the Interdepartmental Committee on the Rehabilitation and Resettlement of Disabled Persons recommended that 'the supplying, at the public expense but on a recoverable basis' of artificial hearing aids should be considered by the then Ministers of Health and Pensions. This recommendation was adopted and Medresco (Medical Research Council) hearing aids, designed by the Post Office, were first issued under the NHS Act in 1947. Specifications for hearing aids are now prepared by the DHSS Advisory Committee on Audiological Equipment. For children, the range of government hearing aids is supplemented by some six commercial aids available under 'call-off' arrangements made with the suppliers by the DHSS. Since 1 July 1980 any individual who cannot be adequately catered for by the NHS range of aids may, at the discretion of the health authority, be fitted with a commercial aid or with two aids if the otologist considers these measures to be desirable.

While services and facilities available for hearing impaired persons under the NHS are prima facie good, a sub-committee of the now disbanded DHSS Advisory Committee on Services for Hearing Impaired People reported in 1975 that:

We should like to place on record our deep concern at the extent to which rehabilitation services for the hearing impaired are lacking in the DHSS. It is barely credible that in the affluent society in which we have lived during the past twenty-five years, so little has been done.[1]

The creation of three new professional groups within the

NHS, audiological scientists (1975), audiological physicians (1975) and hearing therapists (1979) aims, as Stephens[2] says, at providing 'a more comprehensive and effective service for the hearing impaired who have been previously neglected as compared with other handicapped groups'.

Social security

Important social security provision includes attendance allowance, invalidity benefit and benefit in respect of industrial injury.

Attendance Allowance. The Social Security Act 1975 (section 35) and the Social Security (Attendance Allowance) Regulations make provision for payment of a weekly non-contribution allowance to disabled persons who require frequent attention and who satisfy certain conditions as to residence.

To be eligible the claimant must satisfy and have satisfied for the previous six months either or both of the following conditions:

1 He is so severely disabled physically or mentally that he requires:
   (a) frequent attention throughout the day in connection with his bodily functions, or
   (b) continual supervision throughout the day in order to avoid substantial danger to himself or to others.
2 He is so severely disabled physically or mentally that he requires:
   (a) prolonged or repeated attention during the night in connection with his bodily functions, or
   (b) continued supervision throughout the night in order to avoid substantial danger to himself or others.

A person who requires attendance both by day and night will receive a higher allowance; a lower rate is payable to a person satisfying only one of the conditions specified above.

Attendance allowance is not payable in respect of a child under the age of 2. An allowance is payable in respect of a child between 2 and 16 years who, in addition to satisfying the general medical conditions, requires attention substantially in excess of that normally required by a child of the same age and sex.

Invalidity Benefit. The Social Security Act 1975 (section 15) provides for the payment of an invalidity pension and, in certain circumstances, an additional invalidity allowance to a person who has been entitled to sickness benefit and/or a maternity allowance for a period of 168 days (excluding Sundays) and whose incapacity for work continues. A non-contributory invalidity pension may be payable to those not qualifying for contributory benefit. 'Incapacity for work' means to be incapable of work which the person could reasonably be expected to do by reason of some specific disease or bodily or mental disablement.

Industrial injury. The Social Security Act 1975 consolidated, *inter alia*, the National Insurance (Industrial Injuries) Acts 1965–1974 which had themselves consolidated or amended the earlier legislation as to the payment of special national insurance benefits for industrial injuries and prescribed diseases. Occupational deafness, in certain stringently defined circumstances, is a prescribed disease for the purpose of industrial injuries benefits. Occupational deafness is defined as:

Substantial permanent sensorineural hearing loss amounting to at least 50 dB in each ear, being due in the case of at least one ear to occupational noise, and being the average of pure tone losses measured by audiometry over the one, two and three K frequency.

The nature of the occupations in respect of which occupational deafness is a prescribed disease are set out in the Social Security (Industrial Injuries) (Prescribed Diseases) Regulations 1980 (377). The Regulations are complex and should be consulted but, in general, they provide that the extent of disablement in respect of occupational deafness shall be assessed at the lower limit of 20 per cent where the hearing loss in each ear amounts to 50 dB and at an upper limit of 100 per cent where the hearing loss in each ear amounts to 110 dB measured as prescribed above.

The significance of a 'prescribed disease' is that if an impairment such as occupational deafness develops after the claimant has been in one of the listed occupations for a stipulated minimum period the impairment is presumed to have resulted from the employment unless the contrary is proved. It may, for example, with older persons be difficult to distinguish occupational deafness from presbyacusis.

Where a claimant has not been in one of the listed occupations he or she will not be entitled to national insurance 'cover' unless the hearing loss can be shown to be the result of an 'accident arising out of and in the cause of employment' within the scope of section 50 of the Act. An 'accident' can consist of one or more identifiable occasions but is not a gradual process.

Social services

Three statutes, the National Assistance Act 1948, the Chronically Sick and Disabled Persons Act 1970 and the Rating (Disabled Person) Act 1970 and the Disabled Persons Act 1981 contain provisions of importance to hearing impaired people.

The National Assistance Act 1948 (section 29) empowered the then County and County Borough Councils to make arrangements for

Promoting the welfare of persons who are blind, deaf or dumb and other persons who are substantially handicapped by illness, injury and congenital deformity and such other disabilities as may be presecribed by the Minister.

The wording of the Act is 'deaf *or* dumb' not 'deaf *and* dumb' and the word 'deaf' is therefore a generic term covering all categories of hearing impairment. In 1948 local authorities had discretion to provide services for categories of handicapped persons other than the blind and it was not until 1960 that local authority services for the deaf were made mandatory.

Meanwhile, in 1951, a Circular (32/51) had been issued containing a model scheme detailing the services for the deaf or dumb that a local authority must or might provide. This Circular has not been withdrawn and under the Local Government Act 1972 (section 195(3)) schemes approved under the National Assistance Act may pass to new local authorities created as a result of the re-organisation of local government.

The model scheme is applicable both to the deaf and the hard of hearing and the Minister stated that he would be reluctant to approve schemes submitted by local authorities unless they included arrangements for the following services:

1 Assistance to deaf or dumb persons to overcome the effect of their disabilities and to obtain treatment.
2 An advisory service on personal and other problems.
3 Encouragement to deaf or dumb persons to take part in social activities.
4 Visitation by voluntary workers.
   Discretionary services included:
1 Provision of practical assistance in the home.
2 Provision of assistance in obtaining wireless, library and other recreational facilities.
3 Provision of lectures, games and other recreational facilities

in social centres by way of outings, etc.

4 Provision of, or arranging for, special religious services.

5 Provision of travelling facilities so that deaf or dumb persons can take advantage of the service provided.

6 Helping deaf or dumb persons to take holidays at holiday homes.

7 Provision of social centres or holiday homes.

Circular 32/51 also required local authorities to keep a register of handicapped persons who applied for help. Three categories of hearing impairment are specified: deaf without speech; deaf with speech and hard of hearing. The definitions for each of these categories are given in Chapter 1.

Local authorities may carry out their responsibilities to the deaf either by a directly provided service or use the services of a voluntary welfare society for the deaf on an agency basis. Since the passing of the *Local Authority Social Services Act 1970* an increasing number of local authorities have appointed specialist welfare officers for the deaf or hearing impaired. Others have partial agency agreements by which welfare needs are catered for by the social services department leaving welfare and spiritual provision to a voluntary society. While workers in social service departments rely on the referral of hearing impaired persons by colleagues, voluntary societies have a higher incidence of self-referrals. This distinction may be due to several factors. Often, the voluntary society has been long-established and is easily identified as a source of help. Usually a deaf person can go to the social club connected with a voluntary society and introduce himself in an informal way rather than having to go to an office and speak to a receptionist who may not be able to communicate with a profoundly deaf person. Sometimes the office of a local authority social worker for the deaf is not easily accessible to deaf persons in the area served.

There are wide variations in the range and quality of services provided by local authorities. Some authorities do relatively little for the deafened and hard of hearing. Others provide very comprehensive services. The services provided by the Lancashire County Council are based on two fundamental principles. Firstly, that services are provided for all categories of hearing impaired persons and their families including hearing impaired children, the deafened and the deaf-blind. Secondly that all personnel in the social services department should be encouraged to offer their skills and services to the hearing impaired calling on the Authority's social workers for the deaf when specialised help is required.

The Chronically Sick and Disabled Persons Act 1970. Section 2 of this Act requires social services departments, when they are satisfied of the necessity to do so, to provide or give assistance to handicapped persons to obtain any or all of the following services:

1   Practical assistance in the home, wireless, television, library or similar recreational facilities in the home.
2   Recreational and travelling facilities outside the home and assistance in taking advantage of educational facilities.
3   Support in minimising the social and personal consequences of illness and disability to individuals and families.
4   Assistance in carrying out adaptations to the home or provision of additional facilities to secure greater safety, comfort or convenience.
5   Facilities for the taking of holidays.
6   Meals at home or elsewhere.
7   Telephone and any special equipment for its use.

Sections 1 and 2 of the Act also state that:

It shall be the duty of every local authority having functions under Section 29 of the National Assistance Act to inform themselves of the number of persons to whom that section applies within their area and of the need for the making by the authority of arrangements under that section for such persons.

Section 24 of the Act provides that:

The Secretary of State shall collate and present evidence to the Medical Research Council on the need for an institute of hearing research, such institute to have the general function of co-ordinating and promoting research on hearing and assistance to the deaf and hearing.

The Institute was established in 1976 and is based at the University of Nottingham. Clinical outstations have been established at Nottingham and Southampton with Scottish and Welsh sections associated respectively with the Southern General Hospital and the University Hospital of Wales. The initial statement of aims of the Institute included:

1   Investigation of the epidemiology, aetiology, prognosis and clinical description of the various forms of sensorineural hearing loss.

2   Study of the perception of speech in various disorders.
3   Determination of the best set of characteristics for the next generation of hearing aids.
4   The optimisation of speech-reading techniques.
5   The effect of acute auditory failure on speech production.
6   Study of the adaptation of the hearing impaired to their handicap.[3]

The Rating (Disabled Person) Act 1978. This Act enables local authorities to give rate relief to both personal premises and other establishments with facilities for disabled persons. Section 8 of the Act states that 'disabled person' means 'any person who is blind, deaf or dumb or who suffers . . . from any other disability for the time being prescribed for the purposes of Section 29(1) of the National Assistance Act (1948)'.

The Disabled Persons Act 1981 imposes a duty on planning authorities in England and Wales to draw the attention of persons to whom they grant planning permission to certain statutory and other provisions relating to access by disabled persons to buildings and other premises used by the public. 'Other provisions' include reference to the British Standards Institution Code of Practice BS5810 1979 which, *inter alia*, provides that 'selected telephone receivers for public use . . . should be equipped with amplifiers for the benefit of people with impaired hearing.'

Voluntary provision

Both educational and welfare provision for the hearing impaired were pioneered by voluntary effort. The list in Appendix 3 shows that there are many organisations for the hearing impaired operating at local, regional, national and indeed, international level. The activities of some of these have been referred to in earlier chapters and it would be impracticable to attempt more than a brief description of the four national organisations: the Royal National Institute for the Deaf; The British Association of the Hard of Hearing; The British Deaf Association; and The National Deaf Children's Society.

The Royal National Institute for the Deaf

The RNID, founded in 1911 as the National Bureau for Promoting the General Welfare of the Deaf, is the only national body dealing with all aspects of hearing impairment. Through its influential contacts with government departments and pressure group activities it promotes and protects the interests of all the deaf and hard of hearing. It also acts as a co-ordinating agency for organisations interested in various aspects of hearing impairment. The Institute's Council includes representatives from medicine, education and the social services as well as people with other special interests relating to deafness. Representatives of appropriate government departments attend the Institute's Council meetings as observers.

The work of the Institute, as it affects the individual deaf or hard of hearing person or others concerned with the handicap, is divided into four main sections.

Library and information services. The library comprises the most comprehensive collection of books and journals in the world on auditory and associated fields. The information service deals with requests for special information relating to all aspects of hearing and deafness.

Publications. The Institute publishes a range of more than 50 booklets and pamphlets on the medical, technical and social aspects of hearing impairment.

Social services. Advice, support and information are provided on personal, family and employment problems arising from hearing loss. Schemes have been inaugurated to provide television for the deaf and hearing dogs to offer companionship and become the ears of deaf people who live alone. Three residential centres are maintained, catering for deaf people with personal, social problems, disadvantaged deaf young men, deaf blind young people and deaf people of working age. The RNID's homes provide comfortable accommodation for deaf people needing special care and attention.

Research and development. Both medical and technical research are undertaken and sponsored. At the time of writing the programme of medical research includes tinnitus, Ménière's disease, vertigo in the elderly and hearing detection in premature babies. Laboratories are maintained in London and Glasgow for technical research into hearing aids, other special aids to hearing and educational equipment.

The British Association of the Hard of Hearing

The BAHOH, founded in 1947, is the national body for those

who have become wholly or partially deaf usually in post-school life. Its members, therefore, have normal speech and education and employ hearing aids and speech-reading as their means of communication. The Association offers the hard of hearing a range of services, especially facilities for social activities and assistance with personal problems. Social activities are based primarily on more than 200 hard of hearing clubs located throughout the country. The Association arranges holidays both at home and abroad, social gatherings or rallies and weekend courses of lectures and recreational work. Pen-circles are also organised for the lonely or housebound and people who live too far from a club.

Help with personal problems includes advice on hearing aids and employment. Employment advice can be obtained from an experienced vocational officer. In addition, the Association has a team of voluntary social service advisers who can visit individuals to discuss problems and suggest further sources of help. Like all the national organisations for the hearing impaired, the BAHOH maintains close relationships with appropriate government departments to whom complaints and other enquiries can be conveyed.

The British Deaf Association

The BDA, founded in 1890 as the British Deaf and Dumb Association, offers its services to all hearing impaired people although it is primarily the national organisation for those born with severe deafness or those deafened in childhood. There are more than 100 BDA branches, most of them associated with local voluntary centres for adult deaf persons. The BDA undertakes for the deaf many of the activities provided by the BAHOH for the hard of hearing. It organises courses for deaf people of all ages, awards scholarships for higher education and makes grants to assist deaf people in special need. The BDA is Great Britain's representative to the World Federation of the Deaf and studies current international developments in health, education and welfare.

The National Deaf Children's Society

The NDCS was formed in 1944 and is the national organisation concerned with deaf children and their parents. The word 'deaf' in the title is used in its widest sense, applying to all children whose hearing impairment constitutes a handicap. The Society's purpose is to see that children born deaf, or who become deaf at an early age, are enabled to live fulfilling lives. To this end it provides guidance or schooling and further education, a Home Assistant Service for parents and a national holiday scheme. Bursaries are awarded to help train teachers of the deaf and other professionals. Grants are given for medical and technical research and to buy specialised equipment for schools and individual children.

The NDCS works through more than 50 regional associations, some of which have a number of branches.

The Panel of Four

The Panel of Four was established in 1971 following an invitation, from the then Secretary of State for Social Services, to the RNID, BDA, NDCS and BAHOH, to meet him 'to review the field (of services for deaf and hard of hearing people) and to note the matters most apt for further study at an official level with a view to possible further meetings'.

The first discussions with the Secretary of State took place in June 1971 and annual meetings followed with him and, subsequently, the Minister for the Disabled.

It is important to stress that the Panel is not a separately constituted organisation but a permanent forum for the four major national organisations to meet together to discuss issues of common interest. In particular there is clarification of respective policy on many issues where there is no disagreement and on which the Panel can take united action, without infringing upon the specialist services and programmes operated by each of the four.

References

1 DHSS Advisory Committee on Services for Hearing Impaired People. *Report of a Sub-Committee appointed to consider the Rehabilitation of the Adult Hearing Impaired,* September 1975.
2 Stephens, S. D. G. 'The Role of the State in Hearing Health Care', *British Journal of Audiology,* Vol. 16, 1982, p. 259.
3 Anon. 'The Institute of Hearing Research', *Clinical Otolaryngology,* Vol. 3, 1978, pp. 197–198.

Hearing Aid Council
Code of Practice

Whereas the terms of the following Code of Trade Practice have been approved in writing by the Secretary of State for Trade and Industry:

Now, therefore, the Hearing Aid Council, acting pursuant to Section 1(3) of the Hearing Aid Council Act 1968 (hereinafter referred to as 'the Act'), hereby prescribe the following code of trade practice for adoption by persons registered as dispensers of hearing aids under the Act and by persons employing such dispensers:

Dispensers

1 Dispensers shall not indicate the fact that they are registered under the Act by means of any written representation involving the use of words other than 'registered under the Hearing Aid Council Act 1968'.

2 Where those words are employed in an advertisement or promotional literature they shall be accompanied by a statement of the fact that this code of practice is available to any person on request and such a copy shall be made available to anyone requesting it.

3 Dispensers shall maintain at all times a high standard of ethical conduct in the operation of their practice.

4 Dispensers shall at all times give the best possible advice they can to their clients regarding hearing aids and their use.

5 Dispensers shall, where appropriate, make it known to their clients that a hearing aid may not necessarily be of benefit.

6 Dispensers who are not medically qualified shall advise a client to seek medical advice, if he has not already done so, if it appears that the client has been exposed to loud noise in his work or elsewhere or if the client complains of or shows any of the following:

   (a) excessive wax in the ear (whether revealed by examination prior to taking an ear impression or otherwise);
   (b) discharge from the ear;
   (c) dizziness or giddiness (vertigo);
   (d) earache;
   (e) deafness only of short duration or of sudden onset;
   (f) unilateral perceptive deafness;
   (g) conductive hearing loss;
   (h) tinnitus (ringing or other noises in the ear or ears).

7 Dispensers who are not medically qualified shall not:

   (a) represent themselves in any way as being so qualified;
   (b) practise any form of medical or surgical treatment for deafness;
   (c) at any time assume the status of one having surgical or medical knowledge;
   (d) advertise that they are in a position to cure any human failing or physical ill.

8 Dispensers shall not describe themselves as consultants, or specialists, or audiologists unless immediately preceded by the words 'Hearing Aid'.

9 Dispensers shall not designate any premises as a Clinic or Institute.

10 Dispensers shall not interview any potential client at his or her home with regard to the possible provision of a hearing aid unless requested to do so by the client, or unless such client has already been in communication with the dispenser or his employer and, having been given reasonable opportunity, has not indicated objection to such visit.

11 (i) A dispenser must have available for use at every consultation the following equipment:

       (a) A pure tone audiometer (IEC Publication 177 'Pure tone audiometers for general diagnostic purposes'), regularly calibrated to an acceptable standard (BS 2497 Parts 1 to 4), and which contains the facilities for both air and bone conduction audiometry with masking.

(b) An auriscope and specula together with facilities for cleaning them.

(c) Suitable aural impression material and associated equipment.

(d) A range of air conduction (ear-level and body-worn) hearing aids, and of bone conduction hearing aids.

(ii) A dispenser must also be able to arrange speech audiometry when required.

12 Unless a pure tone audiogram taken within the previous two months by, or under the supervision of an ear, nose and throat specialist is available to the dispenser at the time of consultation, appropriate air conduction and bone conduction audiometry must be carried out, with the use of masking where necessary.

13 Before providing or effecting the supply of a hearing aid or before the client has entered into any commitment if this should be later, dispensers shall provide the client in writing with details of:

(i) the conditions relating to any trial, whether free or otherwise;

(ii) the terms of any guarantee;

(iii) the service arrangements available for the hearing aid; and

(iv) the cash price, if any, for the hearing aid and any additional charges and details of any alternative terms or rental terms offered by him to that client.

14 Dispensers shall not take part directly or indirectly in the making of survey enquiries by personal contact or telephone from members of the public regarding deafness or the sale of hearing aids with a view to securing business.

15 Dispensers shall be responsible for the work of any person whose name has been notified to the Registrar in accordance with the provisions of section 3(1) (a) (ii) of the Act and who is operating under their supervision. They shall also ensure that any such person complies with the code of practice for dispensers set out in paragraphs 1 to 14 above.

16 Dispensers who are self-employed or who carry on business in partnership with other dispensers shall comply with the code of practice set out in the preceding paragraphs and also with that part of the code for employers as is set out in

paragraphs 23, 24 and 25 below.
17 The due date by which every dispenser must comply with Rules 11 and 12 is to be 1st December, 1974.

(Reproduced by permission of the Hearing Aid Council)

Hearing impairment scales

A. Social Hearing Handicap Index (Ewertsen/Birk-Nielsen)

1 If you are sitting opposite a person at a distance of about 1 m, will you be able to understand everything if the person speaks in a normal tone of voice? ....
2 Do you have problems in understanding when members of the family are gathered together? ....
3 Is it difficult for you to hear in the kitchen when the water is running? ....
4 Do you find it difficult to hear what the shop assistant says to you? ....
5 Is it difficult for you to carry on a telephone conversation? ....
6 Can you follow the conversation when you are talking to several persons? ....
7 Is it difficult for you to follow a conversation at a tea table with several persons? ....
8 Can you hear most of what is said when sitting at the back of a theatre or a church? ....
9 Can you carry on a conversation with someone sitting at the other end of the room and speaking in a normal tone of voice? ....
10 Can you hear the radio well when it is set at normal volume? ....
11 Can you carry on a conversation easily in a car, tram, train or bus? ....
12 Can you carry on a conversation easily at the dinner table at home? ....
13 Do you understand what is said to you when there is noise from other voices, typewriters, traffic, music? ....
14 Do you recognise a person by his voice? ....
15 Is it difficult for you to hear people speaking on television when it is not turned up? ....
16 Is it difficult for you to follow a conversation at a large dinner table? ....
17 Can you carry on a conversation with someone when the radio or television is not turned up? ....
18 Is it difficult for you to carry on a conversation with someone in a busy street? ....
19 Is it difficult for you to understand what is said to you from an adjoining room? ....
20 Can you carry on a conversation with a person where there is noise, for instance at a restaurant or at a party? ....
21 Do you often misunderstand other people's conversation? ....

B. Scale for Self-assessment of Hearing
(High, Fairbanks, Glorig)

Items for the two forms of the Hearing Handicap Scale[1] are listed
below. The 20 items selected for the first chance half are designated Form A, and the remaining 20 are designated Form B.

Form A

1 If you are 6 to 12ft from the loudspeaker of a radio do you
   understand speech well?
2 Can you carry on a telephone conversation without
   difficulty?
3 If you are 6 to 12ft away from a television set, do you
   understand most of what is said?
4 Can you carry on a conversation with one other person
   when you are on a noisy street corner?
5 Do you hear all right when you are in a street car, airplane,
   bus or train?
6 If there are noises from other voices, typewriters, traffic,
   music, etc., can you understand when someone speaks to
   you?
7 Can you understand a person when you are seated beside
   him and cannot see his face?
8 Can you understand if someone speaks to you while you are
   chewing crisp foods, such as potato chips or celery?
9 Can you carry on a conversation with one other person
   when you are in a noisy place, such as a restaurant or at a
   party?
10 Can you understand if someone speaks to you in a whisper
   and you can't see his face?
11 When you talk with a bus driver, waiter, ticket salesman,
   etc., can you understand all right?
12 Can you carry on a conversation if you are seated across the
   room from someone who speaks in a normal tone of voice?
13 Can you understand women when they talk?
14 Can you carry on a conversation with one other person
   when you are out-of-doors and it is reasonably quiet?
15 When you are in a meeting or at a large dinner table, would
   you know the speaker was talking if you could not see his
   lips moving?
16 Can you follow the conversation when you are at a large

dinner table or in a meeting with a small group?

17   If you are seated under the balcony of a theatre or auditorium, can you hear well enough to follow what is going on?

18   When you are in a large formal gathering (a church, lodge, lecture hall, etc.) can you hear what is said when the speaker *does not* use a microphone?

19   Can you hear the telephone ring when you are in the room where it is located?

20   Can you hear warning signals, such as automobile horns, railway crossing bells, or emergency vehicle sirens?

Form B

1   When you are listening to the radio or watching television, can you hear adequately when the volume is comfortable for most other people?

2   Can you carry on a conversation with one other person when you are travelling in a car with the windows *closed?*

3   Can you carry on a conversation with one other person when you are travelling in a car with the window *open?*

4   Can you carry on a conversation with one other person if there is a radio or television in the same room playing at normal loudness?

5   Can you hear when someone calls to you from another room?

6   Can you understand when someone speaks to you from another room?

7   When you buy something in a shop, do you easily understand the assistant?

8   Can you carry on a conversation with someone who does not speak as loudly as most people?

9   Can you tell if a person is talking when you are seated beside him and cannot see his face?

10   When you ask someone for directions, do you understand what he says?

11   If you are within 3 or 4ft of a person who speaks in a normal tone of voice (assume you are facing one another), can you hear everything he says?

12   Do you recognise the voices of speakers when you don't see them?

13 When you are introduced to someone, can you understand the name the first time it is spoken?
14 Can you hear adequately when you are conversing with more than one person?
15 If you are in an audience, such as in a church or theatre and you are seated near the *front*, can you understand most of what is said?
16 Can you carry on everyday conversations with members of your family without difficulty?
17 If you are in an audience, such as in a church or theatre and you are seated near the *rear*, can you understand most of what is said?
18 When you are in a large formal gathering (a church, lodge, lecture hall, etc.) can you hear what is said when the speaker *does* use a microphone?
19 Can you hear the telephone ring when you are in the next room?
20 Can you hear the night sounds, such as distant trains, bells, dogs barking, trucks passing, and so forth?

[1] Copyright Wallace S. High, Grant Fairbanks, and Aram Glorig, 1964.

C. The Hearing Measurement Scale (Noble and Atherley)

The form of the scale given here is for reference purposes only. *It cannot be used without first reading the instruction manual.* Copies of this and the scale are obtainable from Dr W. G. Noble, Department of Psychology, University of New England, Armidale, NSW 2351, Australia.

Section 1   Speech Hearing

1 (Hh) Do you ever have difficulty hearing in the conversation when you're with one other person when you're at home?
2 (Hh) Do you ever have difficulty hearing in the conversation when you're with one other person outside?
3 (Hm) Do you ever have difficulty in group conversation at home?
4 (Hm) Do you ever have difficulty in group conversation outside?

5 (Hm) Do you ever have difficulty in group conversation at work?

5a[1] (modifier) Is this due to your hearing (retain item 5 score) due to the noise (negate item 5 score) or a bit of both (halve item 5 score)?

6 (Ml) Do you ever have dificulty hearing the speaker at a public gathering?

7 (Hl) Can you always hear what's being said in a television programme?

8 (Hl) Can you always hear what's being said in television news?

9 (Mh) Can you always hear what's being said in a radio programme?

10 (Mh) Can you always hear what's being said in radio news?

11 (Ml) Do you ever have difficulty hearing what's said in a film at the cinema?

Max. Poss. Section Total (76)

[1] Specifically for use among people with chronic acoustic trauma.

Section 2 *Acuity for Non-speech Sound*

12 (Mm) Do you have any pets at home? (Type . . . .) Can you hear it when it . . . . . . (barks, mews, etc.)?

13 (Hl) Can you hear it when someone rings the doorbell or knocks on the door?

14 (Ll) Can you hear a motor horn in the street when you're outside?

15 (Ll) The sound of footsteps outside when you're inside?

16 (Hl) The sound of the door opening when you're inside that room?

17 (Ll) Can you hear the clock ticking in the room?

18 (Lh) The tap running when you turn it on?

19 (Lh) Water boiling in a pan when you're in the kitchen?

Max. Poss. Section Total (28)

Section 3 *Localisation*

20 (Lm) When you hear the sound of people talking and they're in another room would you be able to tell whereabouts this sound was coming from?

21 (Ml) If you're with a group of people and someone you

can't see starts to speak would you be able to tell where that person was sitting?

22 (Mh) If you hear a motor horn or a bell can you always tell which direction it's sounding?

23 (Ml) do you ever turn your head the wrong way when someone calls to you?

24 (Lm) Can you usually tell, from the sound, how far away a person is when he calls to you?

25 (Ml) Have you ever noticed outside that a car you thought, by its sound, was far away turned out to be much closer in fact?

26 (Mh) Outside, do you always move out of the way of something coming up from behind, for instance a car, a trolley or someone walking faster?

Max. Poss. Section Total (28)

Section 4   *Emotional Response*

27 (Mn) Do you think you are more irritable than other people or less so? ('more' scores 5, 'same' and 'less' score 0).

28 (Hl) Do you ever give the wrong answer to someone because you've misheard them?

29 (Mm) When you do this do you treat it lightly or do you get upset?

30 (Hl) How does the other person react? Does he get irritated or make little of it?

31 (Mm) Do you think people are tolerant in this way or do they make fun of you?

32 (Hm) Do you ever get bothered or upset if you are unable to follow a conversation?

33 (Hl) Do you ever get the feeling of being cut off from things because of difficulty in hearing?

33a (modifier) Does this feeling upset you at all? ('yes', add 1 to item 33 score)

Max. Poss. Section Total (45)

Section 5   *Speech Distortion*

34 (Hl) Do you find that people fail to speak clearly?

35 (Mh) What about speakers on television or radio? Do they fail to speak clearly?

36 (Hl) Do you ever have difficulty, in everyday conversa-

tion, understanding what someone is saying even though you can hear what's being said?

Max. Poss. Section Total (20)

Section 6   Tinnitus

37 (Lh) Do you ever get a noise in your ears or in your head? (37a to 37e: A series of items on nature and incidence of tinnitus.)
38 (Hm) Does it ever stop you sleeping?
39 (Mm) Does it upset you?

Max. Poss. Section Total (16)

Section 7   Personal Opinion

40 (Lh) Do you think your hearing is normal?
41 (Lh) Do you think any difficulty with your hearing is particularly serious?
42 (Hl) Does any difficulty with your hearing ever restrict your social life?

Some organisations for hearing impaired

Organisations for the hearing impaired sometimes change their personnel and addresses. To prevent information becoming rapidly out of date only the addresses of the four national organisations referred to in Chapter 11 are given. It is suggested that readers wishing to contact other organisations should obtain the latest addresses from the Information Department of the Royal National Institute for the Deaf.

1 *National organisations*
   (i) Royal National Institute for the Deaf,
        105 Gower Street, London WC1 6AH.
   (ii) British Association of the Hard of Hearing,
        6 Great James Street, London WC1N 3DA.
   (iii) British Deaf Association,
        38 Victoria Place, Carlisle CA1 1EX.
   (iv) National Deaf Children's Society,
        31 Gloucester Place, London W1H 4EA.

2 *Regional associations for the deaf*
   (i) Midland Regional Association for the Deaf
   (ii) North Regional Association for the Deaf
   (iii) Scottish Association for the Deaf
   (iv) South East Regional Association for the Deaf
   (v) Wales Council for the Deaf
   (vi) West Regional Association for the Deaf

3 *Local associations*
   Details of local authority services for hearing impaired people, local voluntary societies for the deaf and clubs for the deaf, can be obtained from the RNID or the BDA, the BAHOH

will provide particulars of local clubs for the hard of hearing
and the NDCS lists of schools and partially hearing units.

4 *Other Organisations for the Hearing Impaired*
Association for Experiment in Deaf Education
Association for the Catholic Deaf of Great Britain and Ireland
Association of Local Voluntary Organisations for the Deaf
Association of Teachers of Lipreading to Adults
Audiology Technicians' Group
Beethoven Fund for Deaf Children
Breakthrough Trust Deaf Hearing Group
British Association of Audiological Physicians
British Association of Otolaryngologists
British Association of Teachers of the Deaf
British Deaf Drivers' Association
British Deaf Ski Club
British Deaf Sports Council
British Sign Language Research Group
British Society of Audiology
British Society of Hearing Therapists
British Sub-Aqua Club Branch 1,000
British Tinnitus Association
Commonwealth Society for the Deaf
Council for the Advancement of Communication with
    Deaf People and the Register of Interpreters
Council for Christian Care
Council for Hearing Impaired Visits and Exchanges
Deaf Broadcasting Campaign
Deaf Christian Fellowship
Deaf Evangelical Fellowship
Deaf-Fax
Deaf Mountaineering Club
Ecumenical Council of Christian Workers with the Deaf
English Deaf Chess Association
Federation of London Deaf Clubs
Friends for the Young Deaf
General Synod of the Church of England Council for the Deaf
Guild of Hearing-Aid Specialists
Hard of Hearing Christian Fellowship
Hearing Aid Council
Hearing Aid Industry Association
Hexham and Newcastle Diocesan Catholic Deaf Service

London Group of Workers with the Deaf
Makaton Vocabulary Development Project
MRC Institute of Hearing Research
The National Association for Deaf/Blind and
    Rubella Handicapped
National Centre for Cued Speech
National Deaf-Blind Helpers' League
National Deaf Children's Sports Association
National Study Group of Further and Higher Education for
    the Hearing Impaired
National Union of the Deaf
Northumbria Workshop with the Deaf
Oto-Rhino Laryngological Research Society (ORS)
Paget Gorman Sign Systems
Project Ear Foundation
Royal Association in Aid of the Deaf and Dumb
Schemes for the Deaf
Society of Hearing Aid Audiologists
Scottish Workshop with the Deaf
Southern Regional Working Party on Signed English
Teachers of Sign Language Group
Westminster & Brentwood Pastoral Service for the Deaf
Yorkshire Workshop with the Deaf

Index

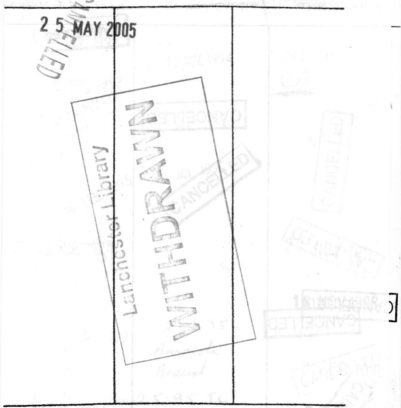